ticked off

ticked off

JANET L. DECESARE

TATE PUBLISHING & *Enterprises*

Published by Tate Publishing & Enterprises, LLC
127 E. Trade Center Terrace | Mustang, Oklahoma 73064 USA
1.888.361.9473 | www.tatepublishing.com

Tate Publishing is committed to excellence in the publishing industry. The company reflects the philosophy established by the founders, based on Psalm 68:11,
"The Lord gave the word and great was the company of those who published it."

Cover design by Lauran Levy
Interior design by Jeff Fisher

Published in the United States of America

ISBN: 978-1-61739-024-1
1. Medical, Diseases, Lyme Disease
2. Biography & Autobiography, Personal Memoirs
10.10.08

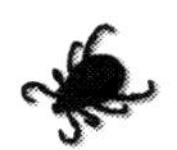

Dedication

In the twelve years of coping and living with Lyme disease, I have met some amazing people. I have spoken to many of you Lyme disease victims either by phone or by e-mail, and we have all become a second family.

This is a dedication to all Lyme disease victims and their families. I pray that my struggles will inspire you, give you courage to not give up; we will prevail in the end!

There are cases where Lyme disease victims have already died. Many of you are suffering and have suffered, many are too weak to take a stand, many are afraid to voice concerns and anger. I am here to speak in your behalf.

I pray that God will continue to bless all of us and our future. We can change history and make a difference.

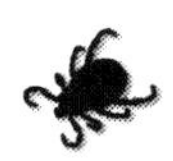

Acknowledgements

People that I owe an unbelievable gratitude to:

Most of all I want to thank God for giving me life, for giving me a brain, two hands, a loving heart, and the know-how to create this book. I could have never lasted this long without your help.

Dr. J, my Lyme disease doctor, you saved my life; how do I repay you for this? I can't say enough for what you have done for me. I am eternally grateful for your individualized attention on how you treated Lyme disease, your knowledge of this insidious disease, and in knowing what Rocky Mounted Spotted Fever looked like. All the previous doctors had no clue what the spots on my shins were.

I am grateful and thankful for what you have done and what you continue to do for me as of 2010. I also thank you for your influence on my journaling for the past twelve years. Who would have ever guessed that my journey with Lyme disease and Rocky Mt. Spotted Fever would become a book?

Dr. S, my Naturopathic doctor. I've never been in a doctor's office like this one. You are like no other doctor I have ever met. You show compassion, caring, are extremely knowledgeable, and have a passion for treating patients with an individualized sense of health care. Dr. S, you have continued to keep striving in taking extra steps in treating my Lyme disease, and I am grateful for this. You taught me how to be in control of my own health care, and I thank you for that.

I have met some beautiful, supportive individuals at Dr. S's office. Although I can't name all of you, I am sure you will know who you are when you read this book. You have helped me by your kind words, encouragement, and compassion. You have given me a sense of well being. We are like one big family there at Dr. S's office, sharing, caring, laughing, and making my journey with Lyme disease a bit more bearable.

Friends, business associates, and sailing buddies of my husband, David, you have shown your interest and kind words on my recovery efforts, and I thank you for caring.

To my Lyme disease buddies, I thank you for your friendship, the many hours we spent at support group meetings, e-mailing each other, telephone conversations, and meeting face-to-face. I know your pain and struggles living with Lyme disease and how we have helped each other by working through them.

My medical doctor, Dr. L., for standing by me trying to understand the complexities of Lyme disease and offering assistance when I need it. You have helped make my journey to move forward and to make a difference.

To my family, who has stood by me with encouraging words and prayers, I thank you.

To my dear friend Carole, you have been my mentor throughout this journey with Lyme disease. You have taught me so much about life, relationships, the love of Jesus, and what it means to be a true friend.

To my daughters, Carrie and Corinne, you have given me the courage to stand up, to fight for life; you have helped me grow in ways that have made me the woman I am today. I also am blessed because I have a son-in-law, Troy, who has joined our family, and now I have another beautiful reason to keep going. Then you, Carrie and Troy, gave me a granddaughter, Monet. What more can I say? I have enjoyed her immensely; she's keeping me "young at heart," and I love her dearly as I do with all of you.

To the most important individual in my life—my husband, David. My words will never be able to express the love and devotion that you have shown me for the past thirty-five years. I know the last twelve years have not been easy for you. I know you have lost many a good night's sleep worrying about me. You have been my "rock" that has weathered many storms. You have put up with my many moods, my anguish, my temper, and my pain, always supporting and loving me throughout this ordeal.

I also owe a deep gratitude to all the people at Tate Publishing, who helped by reading and editing to steer me into the right direction to help create a beautiful book on Lyme disease. May God bless all of you!

WORDS OF WISDOM

Live, love, and dream.

Give thanks to God, for he is walking beside us every day!

Do not let illness destroy your zest for life, lift up thine eyes to the heavens and say thank you for giving you life.

Be a positive influence for others, smiling, laughing, and sharing can make your life much more rewarding; it has for me, and it can work for you.

I never dreamed my life would amount to a "hill of beans." Boy was I surprised.

We only go around this circle called life once, so enjoy the ride!

I can't do much, but what I can do, I put my heart and soul into!

Time is not measured by seconds, minutes, or even hours but how we choose to live our lives!

We have so many things to be grateful for!

Give generously from the heart without thought of a return.

Your attitude can affect your recovery from any illness; how you choose to look at the detours in your life can either strengthen you or deplete your energy and recovery. I chose to think positively, and I have grown into a much stronger person because of it!

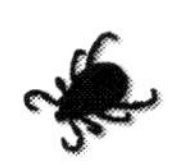

Table of Contents

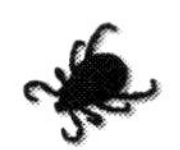

Foreword

There appears to be this something that all of us seek. You can pursue it; however, no one may ever achieve or reach it. On the one end of the spectrum is despair and fear, while at the other end is mere absence.

Why do we seek something that is so hard to obtain? What is the purpose of our pursuit? It is a wise person who understands this journey and the reasons for which we embark upon it. Understanding, patience, and wisdom are the tools you will need if you are only to perceive that you may succeed.

In the beginning, you were unaware of such a thing as predetermination. You could not realize what had been thrust upon you; you had no say. Although you were not in control, your absence did not resolve you from suffering the consequences.

However, you realized that your actions have become more and more important. Maybe more so than anything else. Sure there were things inflicted upon you. You were simply along for the ride, right? You did not realize what was happening. Eventually, reality became apparent. Things had changed. Who can you blame? Where do you turn? Who can you trust? What is the truth?

You are in control, right? You know what happened, don't you? What happened, anyway? Do you really know? Do you understand how you got here? Do you know how you are getting there? Are you prepared for the journey? Realize that the way you answer these questions will determine the quality of the rest of your life.

To obtain your answers, you must hear Janet's story. You need to experience this story. Not to simply pick up a few tips for yourself but to learn how you can survive what is ahead for you. You have a life to live. You might not realize what you have already learned. Janet will help you understand in a charming yet heart-wrenching reality. Janet has a wonderful story. You will love her tales. She has lived and learned along the way, developing the tools necessary to live. Lyme disease does not have Janet; she has it!

You see, this is your journey. It is your life. Open your eyes to what is ahead. Do not be fooled into believing in a destination. Your life is a spectrum. Wherein at one end is optimal health and at the other is illness and disease. And along our pathway we will fluctuate within this spectrum. The traveler who lacks understanding, knowledge, and wisdom will lose their way and hope. Despair not, for you may find your journey begins within.

—William Schneider D.C., FIAMA, Dipl. Ac.

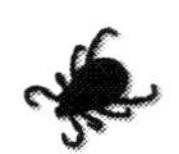

Introduction

I am compelled to write this book about Lyme disease and other tick-borne diseases because I have this dreadful, heart-wrenching disease and have lived with it for twelve years. I am hoping that my story of the struggles that I encountered will inspire other Lyme disease victims and their caregivers (families) to not give up, to keep searching for a Lyme-literate doctor, to keep learning, to research methods of treatment protocols, and to find a cure.

No one really understands what we "Lymies" go through on a daily basis. It is difficult enough to deal with physicians who are not Lyme-literate, who themselves do not fully understand the complexities of Lyme disease and then do not run the appropriate tests to determine what we may have.

Many mistakenly believe that if you are given a simple blood test, this will determine if you have Lyme disease. The problem with this is that many patients never get a positive reading and many have had to rely upon their symptoms.

My story will illustrate the poor knowledge of the treatment of Lyme disease and other tick-borne pathogens. The medical community needs to be educated about these diseases. Lyme disease patients need to be protected from insurance carriers and the state medical boards who do not understand the seriousness of these diseases. But we need to "protect our Lyme-literate physicians" who do understand how serious and how complex these diseases are. It can take months and even years of treatment in order to get the disease under control, if at all.

Our mainstream medical community wants to further ignore how long we patients need to take the only medication available, the antibiotic. They feel the long-term usage is dangerous. Well, maybe it is to a point, but for me and countless of others, using antibiotics is our only solution right now.

Lyme disease is a very debilitating disease, particularly when it becomes chronic.

For example, I am unable to hold a job down; my life has changed drastically throughout this ordeal. I went four and a half years before I was diagnosed, and it may have been longer; I don't know because there are no tests to determine how long I have had Lyme disease. I also have Rocky Mt. Spotted Fever, another tick-borne disease.

Due to the fact that I am still ill with Lyme disease, this book was a long, difficult process. It's hard for me to keep my thoughts together, and you, the reader, should understand the complexities of the disease and how it has infected my mind and thought processes while I struggled to put my experiences into words.

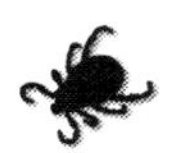

An Invisible Disease:

IT BEGAN IN THE GARDEN

In 1995 I was working in my garden, and I always gardened in my bare feet. We had many deer that roamed all over our property, and they always would feast on my vegetables. I tried different types of deer deterrents to try and keep them out of my garden. I would mix one dozen eggs and water and put it in my sprayer and soak my plants to the point of runoff.

The deer really loved my green beans; I had canned all I needed, and I told my sister to come over and pick what she wanted the next day. So when she arrived, she went outside to the garden; the next thing I knew she was calling me, "Janet, where's all the green beans?" I said, "Silly girl, there were bunches of them last night!" So when I walked out to the garden and started looking around, there were hoof prints all through my vegetable patch, and it looked like someone went down through the garden with an electric knife;

they were sheared off, and all my beautiful, delicious, blue lake green beans were gone. We stood there and laughed!

Although I still get a rush when I see deer meandering onto my property, I've learned to be very cautious. I've even hung Irish Spring soap, push a thin piece of wire through it, and hung it in surrounding trees or on the bushes. The strong aroma sends the deer a message that humans are near. I've also taken dog hair and human hair and sprinkled it around the garden's perimeter; they won't bother there either.

I developed a round, scaly spot on my right foot. It was a round shaped ring with a center, red and itchy. I nearly drove myself crazy from itching it until I bled. I thought it was just poison ivy from being out in the woods and fields around my house with the dogs. When I went in to see Dr. D, he diagnosed and treated me for ringworm. This is when my troubles began. Dr. D prescribed a topical cream to rub on my foot. Then my health took a downward spiral, I was ill constantly. I had numerous infections, bronchitis, pneumonia, and I was unable to concentrate.

The rash I had on my foot was turning a darker red and angry looking. When I returned to Dr. D, he'd just laugh and make a joke about it. "We'll see you next month, because you will be in here sick again!" He would then pat me on my back. I guess he was trying to reassure me. This comment from a professional doctor wasn't too smart. Then his next comment was, "You women just have to have something wrong!" I wasn't getting any better. I was getting worse!

I should have found another doctor when I was seeing Dr. D. His comments were rude and uncalled for. I guess at that time I was just naïve, and I trusted him with my healthcare. I would always ask him, "Why do you make these nasty comments to me?" And he would always reassure me and then apologize. But when I would return to Dr. D.'s office, he would start with the "smart remarks" again. I guess back then I was tired, I wasn't myself because I didn't feel well for a long time, and I didn't want the hassle of locating another doctor at that time. I think I was in a situation where I didn't know any better, and I was sick and tired just wanting someone to help me.

My bones and muscles would ache and burn to the point where I couldn't stand to be up on my feet. I couldn't sit down. I couldn't lay down or even walk. Here I go again back to Dr. D and told him what I was experiencing, and he informed me, Well, I believe you have Chronic Fatigue Syndrome."

Wow, I thought, *finally a diagnosis.* A light at the end of a tunnel? Not so! When my insurance company found this out they went berserk. My insurance company started to increase my premiums. I was already paying $349 a month, $1500 deductible, when my premiums started to climb from that time on. They went from $349 to $401, $469, $601 and $715, it was repulsive how my insurance company treated me from that time forward.

My health wasn't improving. I was slowly deteriorating. My doctor was also a chiropractor who would work occasionally on my back and legs, twisting me like a pretzel. He was trying to alleviate the pain I had in my lower back and the pain that generated down into my legs. This protocol helped for the time being and controlled the pain for brief moments until the pain would hit me, and I nearly collapsed from it.

I will never forget how my brother, Doyle, who has since died, would warn me about letting Dr. D twist me like a pretzel. He would tell me, "Sis, you had better be careful, or Dr. D is going to cause you more harm." He certainly would know he had his share of back problems.

At the time I was doing home healthcare, where I was placed in homes to care for aging parents in their own surroundings. I cared for Alzheimer, cancer, and stroke victims as well as people who were lonely and needed someone to care for them. I finally found a job that I was meant to do, and it was rewarding—not just for me but for the people I cared for. This type of work is not for everyone, and it really takes a great deal of patience, understanding, and fortitude. I fell in love with the majority of my patients, and I knew in my heart that this would become the most rewarding life experience for me.

I shared many wonderful memories with them; we would laugh, I'd read to them, comb their hair, bathed them, dressed them, cooked their meals for them, take them for car rides to buy an ice cream cone or take them shopping. Yes, those were the good ole days. I just wanted them to feel needed and wanted. Every day that came I couldn't wait to see my friends that I was making along the way; it was an awesome experience. While I was caring for my patients and there were times when they were trying to help me, I started slipping backwards again with my health. What in the world was wrong with me and why did I have all this pain and fatigue?

Upon my return to Dr. D, he informed me that he was sending me to see Dr. P, a physiatrist who specialized in muscle and joint problems. When I went into see this doctor he seemed knowledgeable in his field and explained what his treatment protocols would be like. He began using steroid injections on me, and yes, it felt good to be free of the pain. Thank God, I was getting some relief!

He would use heat compresses, ultra sound, and joint injections. "Oh, to be pain free" or so I thought! This was just the tip of the iceberg. I had no idea what was going to happen next.

In 1996 is when I went to work in a hardware store. My job duties consisted of doing inventory, pricing, putting merchandise out on the shelves, lifting boxes, operating cash registers, working in the greenhouse, assisting customers, going up and down stairs to carry merchandise. I started noticing a weight gain, muscle fatigue, joint pains, and my legs would become numb while standing. When I was working I would become so fatigued that I would take my break and find a location in the store where I could sit down and sleep for half an hour. Upon my short nap, I would consume mass amounts of coffee and junk food to keep myself going, I was so exhausted.

I felt as though I was walking around in a fog; my body was here but my mind was elsewhere, but where? This went on for some time. I would get confused over the simplest transactions while working on the register. I couldn't think clearly, I would become agitated with my co-workers, even argumentative at times. I started to not care about doing my job, I just prayed for my shift to be over so I could go home and sleep.

After I arrived home from work, I was dead on my feet! Then I had to come home to my husband, children, big house , a yard, and meals to prepare. There were times when I would be so exhausted at the dinner table that just holding my fork in my hand was all I could do. I wondered why I felt like this and why no one understood what's happening to me.

After all, I was a strong, hard-working woman raising a family, helping my husband with his business, mowing four acres of yard every week, gardening, and holding a job down. I felt like "superwoman." But, as time wore on, so did my health. I thought maybe it was the type of work I was doing and that maybe I needed a change, something less stressful and labor intensive.

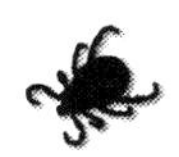

A Ship Without a Sail:

MY UNKNOWN JOURNEY WITH LYME

In 1997 I started working full-time for a temporary clerical service. I worked as a receptionist, computer operator, and as a file clerk in the medical records department.

But, here I go again; I'm just so tired, my feet and legs felt like Jell-O. I found myself making trips to the bathroom for mini naps. I'm almost certain that my employer was getting suspicious as to why I was making so many trips to the bathroom. The office I worked in had a lounge area with a couch. That made it convenient for me to lie down on. I would continue this on and off throughout the day.

Then I noticed an increase in weight gain; this was getting to be a serious problem for me. I always took pride in how I looked and how I dressed while I was working in the office. I made sure my hair was clean, combed, and styled. I dressed professionally and made sure my makeup was just so. But as time wore on, so did I! All this was changing and it was becoming a chore to look good and feel good. I simply did not care about anything! Never realizing the "true reason" was that I was very ill. I would then schedule to visit my doctor again, and—like usual—his comment was, "Janet, you're just working too hard, you're trying to do too much, ease up on yourself, blah, blah, blah," and, as usual, nothing was found to be wrong!

I couldn't wait for 5:00 p.m. so I could clock out and go home. This was my most precious time, so I walked to my car and then fall asleep. Then I'd hear someone tapping on my window asking me, "Why haven't you left the parking lot yet?" I don't know, I must have dozed off. While I was driving home this was becoming another distraction and a deep concern for me. I'd be sitting at a red light, nod off to sleep again, until another person would blow their horn at me.

Many drivers would give me hand gestures, yell out the window at me, "What in the hell's wrong with you?" I wasn't aware that I was doing anything wrong. This went on several times and there were times when I would pull off the road, shut the car off, and go to sleep. When I managed to get home, I had meals to prepare. Thankfully, my girls would start the meals for me and this made life a bit more bearable. As I was eating my dinner, I could barely hold my fork to my mouth because I was so tired. My family would often want to discuss the day's events and I would become despondent, irrational, and even argumentative. I know my family didn't understand me because I couldn't even understand what was happening to me. I was always the jovial one who liked to tell jokes, laugh, and have a good time, but this wasn't the case. Whatever was happening to me was scary, and I was terrified inside this body of mine.

I wasn't sure of myself anymore; I didn't understand why I was acting this way. I decided to try the doctor again so maybe he could shed some light for me. I talked to him and told him of my misfortunes behind the wheel of my car and my attitudes. But, to no avail, was anything accomplished; same old scenario and the same old answers.

The next day, I would be off to work again, just as tired as before. At work, I didn't want to take orders from my supervisors. They would assign me tasks to do and it took me forever to accomplish them. I was argumentative, always defensive, snappy, and couldn't remember what task I was doing. I have to give my employer credit she was extremely patient with me. But why was I having such a difficult time and what in the world was wrong with me?

I couldn't get along with my co-workers and I love everyone: men, women, and children. I can start a conversation with anyone, whether at work, in the grocery store, or the gas station and I love helping people.

There were many days at work when I would just break down and cry, excuse myself, and become so sick to my stomach. Many days I would sit alone at the lunch table, while others sat and stared at me. They probably thought I was some kind of "wacko!"

I was becoming more and more paranoid while I was around people. I couldn't function, I couldn't remember what I was doing, where I was, why I was doing the job that I was trained to do. Nothing was working for me! I suffered in silence for several months. I was too embarrassed to even tell my husband or my family of what I was experiencing, for fear that they would think I was mentally ill, or worse.

One day my supervisor came to me and said, "Janet, I have to let you go!" That was devastating and demeaning to me. I believe I did everything possible to get her to change her mind besides getting down on my knees and beg to keep my job. Now what? I drove around town for hours, stopped at the mall, wandered around, and stopped to get coffee just to keep the energy up to avoid coming home too soon. I couldn't tell my husband and family that I lost my job. So for days, I would get up, get dressed, and drive around town, stopping here and there to fill my time in until it was time to return home. I hated lying to them but I was afraid, embarrassed, and ashamed that I couldn't hold a job.

So I went back to my doctor and told him what had happened and begged him to help me figure out what was wrong with me. I got the same old thing, "You're just tired, maybe you've got some depression coming on board, you need to tell your husband what happened because you're carrying all this guilt around and this is not going to help you in the long run. Let me order you a prescription for anxiety."

Well, I finally decided I had to confess; I told my husband that they let me go because I couldn't function. He wasn't too happy with me, either, so I figured I had more problems and my health took a downfall again.

I found a job as a bank teller, but had the same problems and I could feel my health spiraling out of control again. There were a multitude of items that I was responsible for and I just couldn't handle them, either. There was multi-tasking, I'd argue with the customers, couldn't handle simple transactions, was exhausted, sick to my stomach, eating junk food, and drinking coffee just to keep going. Here we go again: the supervisor would call me into her office. "Janet, I really like you and your co-workers like you, too, but I don't believe this is the job for you." I begged her to let me try again and so she gave me a second chance. But it didn't work; I knew when she called me into her office, I was finished. She was very kind, understanding, and apologetic. I told her, "You don't need to apologize to me, I failed you, I can't do this job, but I do thank you for everything."

I was in a daze; I didn't know where to turn or who to talk to. Why was this happening to me? After a few days, I confessed to my husband again that I failed, I can't hold any job down, and I don't know why!

It was extremely rough; I felt like a stranger in my own family. No one could understand and neither could I as to what was happening to me. With my husband carrying the load financially, it was difficult, to say the least. But what I didn't know was how rough my life would become!

Our biggest concern was our health insurance and there again I had no clue what our future held for us. I failed, I blamed myself I didn't feel like I was holding up my end of the bargain. So we decided that maybe I should take a break for a year. We believed that the doctor was correct with his diagnosis of depression.

Our oldest daughter was planning a wedding in 1998. We had a huge garden and yard that I managed to take care of. I had to prove to myself and my husband that I was capable of doing something right for a change.

Hosting the wedding there would be plenty of work and I knew I could handle this. What with all the baking to do, invitations, showers, and knowing I'm good at this, I was excited—I found something I could do.

My health continued to decline. In the months following the wedding, I developed spots on my shins, respiratory problems, malaise, headaches, chills, and fevers. But I kept going; after all, I was getting ready for a wedding. There was no doubt that the wedding pushed me beyond my limits, but it was well worth the time invested. I had a wonderful time, even at the reception. I danced my legs off and felt like I could drop over at any given moment.

As time wore on, so did my health!

I tried to work at another home health care agency but was unable to do so due to the same health issues as before. This meant that I had to stay home and recover before I could go back to my patients. I rested, took my medicines, recovered, and went back to caring for my friends. I was happy too see them as much as they were to see me. We had a lot of catching up to do. When my patients would take a nap, so would I. I could feel the life being slowly drained away from me once again. My weight shot up another ten pounds; of course, could this be from all the goodies that I would prepare for my patients and the thoughtfulness of their loved ones who would leave yummies there for us to eat?

The doctor and my husband felt that I needed to give up taking care of my patients for a while. They felt that I needed the rest and time for my body to heal. So I spoke to my employer and I told my patients that I needed to take a furlough. They were saddened; my employer was very understanding and told me, "You will be missed dearly!" This just about broke my heart because I felt sad for leaving, but I was in no condition to care for anyone else. I've worked in many types of jobs, but none of them gave me the satisfaction that I earned while caring for them. I only knew that I would miss them as well and prayed that someday soon, I would get the opportunity to care for them again.

While on furlough, I was starting to have panic attacks, nervousness, and the anxiety was overwhelming for me at times. I figured it was probably just the depression that the doctor discussed with me. I made an appointment with Dr. P., who sent me for x-rays of my back which revealed I had a pinched nerve, disks were disintegrating, spurs and arthritis affected my spinal column. He immediately prescribed anti-inflammatory and pain pills. By this time, I was so discouraged and I didn't know what to do or what to think. I constantly prayed to God but to no avail; prayers didn't seem to be heard.

My doctor then sent me to see an Endocrinologist, Dr. J, who felt that maybe my thyroid was the problem now. My weight continued to climb and I started developing sore throats and swollen glands. Dr. J ran some tests to check on my thyroid. As usual, tests came back normal and he told me it was depression. I took his word and continued on with my life as best as I could. I dieted, exercised, and was starting to regain my strength once again. This didn't last for long until my health spiraled out of control again.

I wasn't getting any results from the past doctors so I decided to start "doctor shopping" to find someone else who may be able to help find the problem with me. I went to the next doctor, Dr. W. I hoped maybe an older, more experienced doctor could help me figure out this dilemma I was facing. We talked about everything that I had been experiencing sorted through all my medical records, test results, and findings. He did his own testing and informed me, "You do not have Chronic Fatigue. It was a misdiagnosis; I'm so sorry for what you have been through." He then informed me, "I will write a letter to your insurance company and inform them of this mistake." Well, it didn't really matter, because the costs of my insurance didn't change. I asked him if I could go back to work and he said, "I don't see a problem with that." I was so thankful that I finally found someone who was willing to work with me.

I decided to go back to work this time as a nurse's assistant caring for older adults. I went to a local nursing home, filled out the application, and waited for an answer. The nursing home supervisor called me into her office and told me I got the job. I was thrilled to death! Finally, I was going to get the education that I so needed to do this new job adventure. What a day; my husband was thrilled for me as well! The nursing home sent me to another location to begin my training. I studied, watched movies on caring for the elderly, bedside manners, I went on field trips with other state tested nurses for hands-on training. It was wonderful, fun, and I couldn't wait!

I studied until my eyes hurt, my hands would ache and go numb from all the homework assignments, but that didn't matter to me. I was finally on my way back into the workforce and I loved every minute of it. My goal and my potential was finally being met, it was exciting.

Maybe to some people, the thought of cleaning up after a patient or helping someone face their own departure isn't appealing, but to me it was tremendous and rewarding. And of all the patients that I took care of previously, I loved them dearly.

On the day of my final test, my dream job, my husband found me sitting on the steps in our home with what we thought was a heart attack. I had sweaty palms, shortness of breath, chest, and stomach pains. My husband helped me into our car and drove me to the first hospital. All the way there, I was irritable and how I prayed that what was happening to me was just a case of "cold feet" because of the test I was to take. Upon arriving to the hospital, they immediately sent me to the cardiac unit where tests were performed on me. They placed me on a heart monitor and oxygen.

I wondered where my husband was; why couldn't he come back here with me? I kept asking the nurse, he surely was done with the paperwork, so please ask him to come back with me? The poor man, my husband, with what he's had to go through with me is truly amazing. I am such a blessed woman to have him stick by my side throughout this ordeal. I know of many husbands and wives that when they become ill have walked away or just simply can't handle it.

Finally, the nurses let my husband come back to sit with me. They had put me through all the grueling tests. But after they returned me to my room, they just left me lay there in the cardiac unit, no oxygen, no heart monitor, and told me they would check on me later. "Later, what do you mean, later?" I don't remember how long I laid there waiting for a nurse or even a doctor to come in to see me, but no one came. This was ridiculous; my husband was "ticked off," and that's putting it nicely. "Why aren't you doing anything for her?" he would ask. I was so disgusted, I told my husband get my clothes, "I'm getting out of here!" and I did! I proceeded to check out of the hospital, we came home, and I called Dr. W—my family doctor. He was on vacation and his associate, Dr. F, told me to go directly to hospital #2. We drove down and they admitted me where I stayed for other tests. By this time, my husband was so discouraged and distraught I think he thought I was going to die. All we could think about was our insurance or losing our home. I know to some of you that may sound callous, but that's how it is. When you're self-employed, it's not easy, everything is so expensive. We had already spent thousands of dollars on numerous doctors with no answers as to what in the world was wrong with me. We thought doctors were supposed to have the know-how and determine what the patient is dealing with and then fix it. We soon learned that this was going to be a battle.

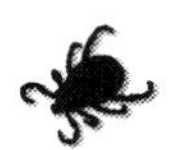

Ticked Off:

WHAT IS LYME DISEASE?

When Lyme disease becomes chronic, other diseases and complications can come along with it. This is because Lyme disease wasn't diagnosed when we were first bitten. Chronic Lyme patients face the lack of prudence as to how long we should be on the antibiotics. In many cases, it's known that some have been on antibiotics for five years and longer and are doing fine. But there are others who can't be on antibiotics for a long period of time.

Lyme disease is the fastest growing infectious disease in America. It should be right on top of the list with AIDS. Lyme disease is the most common tick-borne disease in the United States. It is caused by the spirochete, borellia burgdorferi. It may exist in a chronic form and be the result of either persistent infections by b. burgdorferi, damage caused by the original infectious process, or the presence of co-infection with another organism transmitted by the Ixode ticks. The purpose of this study is to determine the safety and effectiveness, in seronegative patients, of intensive antibiotic treatment in eliminating symptoms of "Chronic Lyme disease."

You become infected when you are bitten by a tick that has fed on an animal (typically a white-tailed deer) that happens to be harboring this bug. More than half of patients with Lyme disease do not know they have been bitten, and first suspect the disease when they develop the signature bull's eye rash. This is sometimes accompanied with flu-like symptoms. The rash usually persists for two to four weeks. This early stage of this disease is the best time to treat it. However, the disease may not be easy to recognize in patients who sometimes never develop the rash. If the disease is missed early on, the infection can involve the joints, the heart, and the brain resulting in a disabling and chronic illness.

What are ticks? Ticks are related to spiders (arachnids) and are the largest of the order (acarina.) The Ixodidae, or hard ticks, feed on the blood of vertebrae animals and carry disease that affect humans.

Deer thrive in forest areas, where there are trees enough to hide in and open land to feed upon. Ticks like the dense shrub; they like moist humidity around 85 degrees, where there's no light down under the leaf litter and thickets.

Some experts believe that when a forest fire happens, it cleans up the tick-infested areas. Some believe that controlled burns would be the most effective to rid the tick populations. We are slowly pushing the deer into our backyards and front yards; their habitat is slowly being taken away due to more and more homes that are being built. The farmlands are being sold out and turned into housing developments. We have curtailed hunting, we aren't able to have controlled burns, we have rodents in our fields, landscaping, and gardens, which are creating a "hot bed" for ticks, their host families, and diseases.

I have read about flagging for ticks by dragging a cloth over an area so ticks can be snagged upon it. The first thing you do is stir up the leaf litter and the second thing is catch the ticks so they can then be studied in a lab for blood diseases.[1]

Your dog has as much a danger of getting this disease as you do. Recent research has shown that dogs may harbor the Lyme disease bacteria and spread the bacteria to previously uninfected ticks, much in the same way deer and mice are known to do. This does not mean you can catch Lyme disease from your dog, just that he or she could be helping spread the disease by infecting new ticks.

I have had many nasty remarks made to me about my dogs and how that's how I caught Lyme disease. Not true. A few family members would make comments about me owning a dog and how they passed it to me. My husband and I have always had a dog or dogs in the house, and I'm not letting this discourage me from owning one. Pets are wonderful, understanding, furry friends; you just need to know the facts and preventative methods on safeguarding your home and yourself.

The clinical symptoms for a dog include arthritis, sudden onset of severe pain and lameness, fever, lethargy, loss of appetite, and depression. Lyme disease also infects their heart, brain, and kidneys. Protect your four-legged friends after they have been outdoors, especially in tall grass, or brush, which is a favorite place for ticks. Brushing your dog's coat after each outing helps.

If a tick is attached to your dog's skin, remove it carefully with tweezers, pulling back steadily and slowly to ease out the tick's mouthparts, wash the area, and your hands. Use baths, dips, and flea and tick collars as recommended. If able to, cut the brush and mow the grass where your dogs play. You can also treat your yard with a vet recommended tick-killing spray. Ask your vet about vaccinating your four-legged friends.[2]

Of course, there are natural alternatives to help control the tick populations. If you live in a rural area, you could purchase guinea hens to roam freely on your property. They love ticks; our neighbor has them and they are always out there roaming around enjoying their feasts and help keep the tick population under control.

In the meantime, we were searching on the internet and a topic on Lyme disease appeared. I thought, "Hmmm, I never heard of that!" When I was working, my older sister who lives in another state knew of a woman who had Lyme disease. We spoke on the phone and I told her my symptoms. We checked the internet website for Lyme disease and found the information about this disease. We couldn't believe all the different sites on this mysterious disease; little did we know what was about to happen.

When I was in the hospital, they too put me through all the grueling tests and, of course, all my results came back normal. What on earth was I dealing with and why couldn't someone figure it out?

Dr. W returned from his vacation and came in to see me; he then ordered for my release and three days later, I was ill again. My body was wracked with pain, fatigue, headaches, stiff neck, joint and muscle pain, numbness, depression, sleep disturbances, stabbing pain, and ringing in my ears. It was a full blown disaster for me and I didn't know what to think or how I felt about all of this. I went back to Dr. W, and he wanted to run some viral tests, gastrointestinal, etc.

When I approached him and asked him to run a Lyme disease test, I thought he would die! He blatantly said, "There's no Lyme disease in Ohio. Why on earth do you think you have Lyme disease?" I begged him, "Please, Doctor, I'm at the mercy of you to help me find out what's wrong with me."

Dr. W proceeded to order up tests and a week and a half later they came back positive. He proceeded to tell me, "I don't know what to do or how to treat you," so he sent me to see an Infectious Doctor, Dr. C. After all the tests were run and we discussed the health problems that I had been dealing with all along this is how it was noted:

> Oct. 28, 1999 First Noted, Pt. had rash, joint & muscle spasms, immobility, extreme fatigue, mental confusion, memory impairment, anxiety attacks, photosensitivity, fevers, parasthesia (transient), bilaterally upper & lower extremities, insomnia, wt. gain, hearing deficit.
>
> Does Pt. Complain Yes, pain and discomfort, sharp, aching joint pain, daily and at prolonged intervals needs to rest, low grade fevers of 102* and under, myalgias, continuous mild to severe depending on activity, intermittent headaches, memory and concentration
>
> Pt. Physical Activities Sitting and Standing–1 hr. causes joint immobility, Walking, Bending, Lifting–2 hrs. limited, Joint pain, Myalgia and fatigue
>
> Handling Objects–Limited—Extremity numbness
>
> Traveling–no more than short car trips
>
> Pt. Symptoms ECM Rash, circular rash on both ankles, CNS–tingling, dizziness, numbness of extremities, short term memory, loss of concentration
>
> Arthritis–Swelling in knees, ankles, feet, hips, arms, fingers and shoulders

Cardio–Shortness of Breath

Bell's Palsy–No

Malaise–Extreme fatigue, Headaches–front and back of Head, Fevers–chills, night sweats, low grade fevers,

Muscle Pain–arms, legs, feet

G.I.–nausea, constipation, wt. gain, abdominal pain

Visual–floaters, Hearing–ringing and stabbing in ears

ENT–sinus drainage

Upon seeing this Infectious Disease Dr. C, two days later I had a nurse, IV technician, and mobile x-ray unit arrive at my home to start treatments. At that time, I was too ill to leave my home and my insurance company was willing to let me be treated in my own surroundings. My husband helped to dress me and I was brought downstairs to the living room to start my treatments. The mobile x-ray technician placed a unit behind my back while the nurse inserted a PICC line in my vein. The reason for this was to carefully insert the line and not to hit the heart. The IV was a Rocephin Drip per twenty days, Amoxicillin 500 mg, twice a day, Zyrtec 10mg once daily, Mega B100 and a multivitamin.

I was on the IV for one and one half weeks when I developed an infection in my arm. The nurse came to remove the PICC line from my right arm. The mobile x-ray tech returned to place another unit behind my back so the nurse could safely insert the line not to hit the heart in my left arm. The nurse returned to remove the PICC line because I developed serum sickness, so I wasn't on the IV for the initial twenty days.

Let me explain what serum sickness is: it's an allergic reaction that occurs days to weeks after an injection of a foreign substance, including fever, skin rash, joint pain, swollen lymph nodes, and occasional kidney problems or protein in the urine[3].

A PICC line is a Peripherally Inserted Central Catheter. It is a long, slender, small, flexible tube that is inserted into a peripheral vein, typically in the upper arm and advanced until the catheter tip terminates in a large vein in your chest near the heart to obtain intravenous access. It's for use of antibiotic treatments for longer lasting methods[4].

I had many discussions with the nurse who came to my home about what to expect with this disease. She was very subtle and told me, "You have a long road ahead of you, dear!"

While I was trying to balance my life and live with my symptoms, we researched on the internet and I found other people who suffered with this disease and contacted them. They told me that after they were on the IV treatment in the beginning, they went on an oral antibiotic. After the IV was removed, we went back to the doctor and he told me, "You're cured!"

"No, doctor, there is no cure for this disease," I said. Aren't you supposed to put me on an oral antibiotic for a while? "No," he said, "you need to go and have tests run for cancer, MS, Lupus, etc." Well, I knew he was wrong, because I had spoken to other Lyme disease patients and other doctors who treat Lyme disease, and they all confirmed that I should be using an oral antibiotic. So we ended up paying the bill off with Dr. C, and we left. Then my health took a downward spiral.

Our insurance company went through the roof when all this took place. After my treatments at home, the insurance company paid out $12,000 for two and a half weeks of treatment.

I went to see Dr. F, who replaced Dr. W when he retired. Oh the joy of it all! Perhaps a younger doctor fresh out of college may be more knowledgeable, we thought.

> On Aug. 10, 1999, Dr. F, Janet, came into my office. She was treated for sixteen days with a Rocephrin IV drip for the diagnosis of Lyme disease based on IgM positive serologies. The pt. had been having symptoms for 3 years after a vacation in a wooded area and because of this strong history, the IgM being positive, I went on and treated her. I aborted therapy at 16 days because of neutropenia and fevers which I suspected was drug and serum sickness. She is back here in my office with a follow-up and I may remind you that she had an elevated sedentary rate and C-reactive protein. On her follow-up visit, she complained of being tired, joint pains, backache, overall lack of attention in terms of her memory and numbness in her extremities.
>
> On August 24, 1999 pt. developed a yeast infection, Monistat was prescribed but did not help, fever over 101*, chills, was in emergency room, vomited, weakness, chest pain.

My husband told the emergency room doctor that I had Lyme disease. His response was, "I don't know anything about Lyme, only from what I've read about in my textbooks." He remarked, "You know more about how the disease works than I do."

> Pt. was worked up by Dr. D, who thought she had Chronic Fatigue, then subsequently made a medical misdiagnosis, in which case had found she had Lyme disease. Indeed she does have IgM's that are positive, with this current set of problems and also I suspect that this is a reasonable diagnosis. As you may know, also the Lyme antibody IgG has at least two of the antibodies positive and the Western Blot IgM is positive, indicating strong evidence for serological identity

> to this organism. She was at the ER due to chest pains, but EKG came back normal.
>
> At this point in time, I suspect that this pt. may have ongoing Lyme disease and I think it is reasonable to treat her for both CNS and Arthritis, also. My pt. lives on a farm, big yard, and gardens.

By this time, I was fit to be tied and my husband was ready to give up! Dr. F felt I should go see a dermatologist at a clinic, so we scheduled an appointment and my husband took time off once again to go and see what he had to say. Dr. F didn't understand what was happening to my skin; it was itching and red nearly all the time.

Dr. L looked at my shins and asked if I had been treated for it? Yes, I said. Dr. L did not know what the red spots on my shins were at the time. He examined me and he looked at my legs down around my shins and made his observations. I thought, being a dermatologist, he would want to do a biopsy of the spots on my shins, but he didn't. He said Dr. L couldn't test my skin accurately because I had already been on antibiotics. He proceeded to leave the examination room after some discussion and returned with a list of doctors who specialized in my various symptoms that I was complaining about. At which time, my husband, David, asked him, "How much do we owe you?" He said $85. We paid the bill and left. One the way home we discussed our next move was to get in touch with some other people who had Lyme disease and find out who they went to. That's when we found Dr. J.

"Geez, why did we even bother to come up here, this is a total waste of time!" I couldn't believe the audacity of this doctor and him not even taking a scraping off my shin to send in for a biopsy. I'll tell you, neither one of us was too thrilled over this visit. My husband and I were extremely discouraged at this point in time. We felt that this doctor didn't understand Lyme disease and the complexities of it.

I came home and went to bed; I was totally exhausted and I hurt all over again. I slowly slipped backwards and my health took another downward spiral. I called my sister and asked if she could find out from the lady she knew of who had Lyme disease, if she could get her doctor's name. We were desperate trying to figure out what the next step was going to be. I called other people in Northeastern Ohio and I also called my sister in Pennsylvania who also helped us unravel the mystery.

I made an appt. with Dr. J, out of state, and this meant my insurance wasn't going to pay for this. We didn't know, but we had to do something because I wasn't improving and the doctors in Ohio weren't helping me.

This doctor was not like most doctors; he had a quaint office, the staff were unbelievably kind and supportive, and then in walked Dr. J. He was remarkable; we introduced ourselves to him, and my husband really took to this doctor. He really liked him and that made the trip there worth it. We discussed all my health problems, showed him test results, x-rays, blood work, and then I showed him my shins. When he examined the spots all over my shins, he knew exactly what he was looking at. He said, "You have had Rocky Mt. Spotted Fever at some point in your life." My husband and I just looked at each other. I think I started to cry; we couldn't believe after seeing all these previous doctors, visiting hospitals, and nothing was ever mentioned of Rocky Mt. Spotted Fever. What in the world? He immediately prescribed oral antibiotics and I started to see a little ray of light because I started to feel better.

I am writing this book to campaign for those who cannot speak for themselves or who are afraid to speak up for themselves.

I am so grateful to Dr. J for what he has done for me. His commitment is commendable to helping his patients, he's knowledgeable, trusting, and I have a great deal of respect for his honesty. Dr. J proceeded to explain to me how Lyme disease works.

Dr. J, my Lyme disease doctor, would tell me be sure to obtain proper rest and avoid becoming overtired! He advised me to take an early afternoon nap before the onset of fatigue and, if possible, before late evening socializing or planned work events.

Herxheimer Reaction is when treatment is begun, you often feel worse before you improve. This usually occurs within the first few days, and may last from several days to several weeks. The best way to deal with this is to sleep as much as possible and use Advil or Tylenol to help you get through it. Depression and irritability can be expected as part of your Herxheimer Reaction. Often you will see a late afternoon, low grade fever in the order of 99–100*.

As treatment progresses, you will improve slowly in a step-like manner. There will be good days and bad days. Keep a diary of your progress to help identify symptoms.

As a follow up, they would like to see you on a monthly basis to check your progress, unless otherwise directed. Long term treatment may require periodic blood testing.

Possible side effects include nausea, vomiting, diarrhea, vaginitis, weakness, headaches, increased frequency of urination, prolonged bleeding from cuts, bruising, and sensitivity to light.

It's important to watch for allergic reactions by looking for danger signals such as respiratory distress (shortness of breath), chest tightness, reddened rashes, and itching.

I was using two antibiotics, Zyrtec for allergies, Buspar for nerves, Diflucan for yeast infections, several herbs, and supplements to maintain a balance for my system.

This disease has affected me in many numerous ways. It has affected my husband, David, probably the worst. He doesn't talk about it much because you can see the hurt and disgust in his eyes. He has such a low tolerance to the medical field for all the past ignorant mistakes that these professional men and women have made. To him, it's inexcusable for the way the medical society has treated his wife!

Having Lyme disease is difficult enough for the victim; for the "caregiver", whether it is your spouse or children, it's terrifying. Who wants to watch a loved one become afflicted with an illness? Besides that, it has to do with all the "hoops" and "political overtones" that we deal with when you have Lyme disease.

I found a support group online in Cleveland, Ohio, with a wonderful group of men and women who also suffer with Lyme disease. My husband and I would attend meetings when possible, but it wasn't always convenient to do. The woman who organized the support group had a newsletter with stories and articles of patients and their personal struggles to get medical help, info on Lyme disease treatments, protocols, legislation, and funny quotes. All of this was targeted to help the patient and their families in letting them know they are not alone in fighting this disease.

I also have written articles on Lyme disease, I have stories and comments on sites on the internet and I campaign as much as possible by writing letters to Congressmen for help. I have spoken to many other doctors in and around the U.S., Canada, and Switzerland who have performed experimental treatments on Lyme disease patients.

We Lyme disease patients have to help ourselves; we have all become expertly trained for what to look for and diagnose our symptoms, because the medical field has not or does not offer much support. They have made us feel like "it's all in our heads" and this is so wrong!

How can a doctor tell the difference between stress, aging, or contracting Lyme? Why do they not test us when we ask to be tested for Lyme disease? Lyme disease never was mentioned in my conversations with the doctors from 1995–1999. I went for four years, if not longer, not knowing what was wrong with me and nothing ever came up in conversation about Lyme disease.

The reasons I never mention the names of my wonderful doctors is for their protection as well as mine. There are doctors who treat Lyme disease in New York, Connecticut, New Jersey, and other states who are being harassed by insurance companies and state medical boards. These doctors are being investigated for conduct on how they treat Lyme disease by using aggressive antibiotics. I will protect my doctor and doctors because they are diligently working in my best interest to make me well again.

I am not intimidated and I am not afraid to speak up anymore when it comes to this disease. There are a great many "Lyme disease warriors" who are taking a stand to get this disease recognized and brought up front to raise awareness and to get Lyme disease the proper recognition it so deserves. This is a real and damaging disease and it's about time that we take a stand and bring it into focus. What kind of future do we have if we can't get the proper diagnosis and the proper treatment?

Antibiotics alleviate the symptoms of disease, but we really don't have a cure for it, yet! In my opinion, the only way we're going to develop effective treatments will be to treat the cause of this disease and not just the symptoms. Many patients have only clinical symptoms and there are forty-six symptoms that they are treated for.

Our blood tests are not accurate enough to determine if a patient has Lyme disease. So we need better, reliable tests to determine this disease. There are certain clues that can alert a physician of the probability of having been exposed to a tick bite.

Everyone wants to say, "You can't get it here in Ohio," and that's not true! The critics state that it only is in certain parts of the U.S. Well, if you think about it, you can leave the state of Ohio and go to Pennsylvania, West Virginia, Indiana, Kentucky, Michigan, and New York in a day's time, and if you are in an endemic area that's prevalent for ticks you can pick it up, come home, and not even know it's on you.

That was my case, twelve years ago. I was working in our garden and I gardened in my bare feet. We have many deer on our property and they were always in my garden eating my veggies. I put out all kinds of deer deterrents to try and keep them out of my area.

I developed a "bulls-eye" rash on my foot and that's when I went to Dr. D, and he treated me for ringworm; this is when all my troubles began! Lyme disease is a whole body disease it affects you from head to toe. Some days are good and some days are bad, you never know what's going too happen or how you will feel.

There was a young lady named Jenny Umphress who died at a young age from Lyme disease. She said to her mother once, "Mom, it is bad enough to be sick and have Lyme disease, but it is worse to have to keep proving it over and over again." Her mother wrote a book called, *Twice an Angel—Living and Dying with Lyme dis-*

ease. It is an excellent true story of the battle with Lyme and what Jenny experienced was a nightmare. She was and still is a crusader for many of us.

But her story and so many countless people know all too well what she went through to get diagnosed. All of us have had to deal with this disease on a constant basis. For some of us, it never lets up! I have decided that no matter what the cost or how much pain I have in my own body, to be a crusader not just for myself but for others who can't speak or who are debilitated and help them in any way possible.

During the week of Feb. 1–10th, my other Lyme disease friend and I decided to run a campaign for Lyme disease. We put up lime green ribbons on the trees throughout my neighborhood and had the newspaper come out and do an article for us. We also created a huge sign to look like a postcard addressed to President Bush. It was called, "Have a Heart, Mr. President" for his help and support in fighting for Lyme disease. Then we had everyone in our support group, friends, and family send a postcard with a green heart or the word "Lyme" written on the outside of the postcard. We sent them to the President; did he receive any of them? I doubt it, we never heard from anyone in Washington.

To top it off, when the newspaper reporter interviewed my friend and me, he treated us rudely! The reporter went to doctors who were not Lyme-literate and the comments that were made from these doctors made us look like "incompetent jokesters." He treated us as though we didn't know what we were talking about. I know this upset my friend deeply; it didn't upset me because I'm aware of how the media and most "mainstream medical" look at us Lyme patients. That's why it is so aggravating when we try to campaign or raise awareness; they turn on us, it's not fair! Somewhere in time, they have got to listen to us!

We Lyme disease patients deserve fair and proper treatment. It is an ongoing struggle: emotionally, physically, mentally, and financially. Leave our literate Lyme disease doctors alone who treat long-term chronic patients. Let them do their job. We do not have any other medications to try other than the antibiotic. If you want our doctor's to stop using antibiotics, then why don't you get busy and create a drug for us to use? Even clinical trial studies for us chronic patients could give us some hope for a healthier future.

The other controversy right now over chronic Lyme disease is among The Medical Conduct Boards, The Infectious Disease Society, and the Insurance Companies. The stipulations that they are placing on chronic Lyme sufferers is unjust! They are putting stipulations on patients, telling us, "If you never had a tell-tale bulls' eye rash or at least two positive blood tests, we won't cover the patient." This is so wrong!

Yes, it is true that many Lyme patients have not seen or knew they had a rash, and all they had to go on were clinical symptoms and sometimes the doctor can't get a positive reading for Lyme. I think it's high time for us to have reliable tests to determine if it's Lyme disease or other tick-borne diseases. If we had knowledgeable doctors who knew what to look for, maybe we all wouldn't be in the mess we're in.

The above mentioned are tearing our literate Lyme disease doctors away from patients with long term usage of the antibiotics. Some of the "mainstream medical community" think that if you use the IV drip for twenty days up to four weeks, that's ample enough time to put the disease under control. If you continue to have other problems, it's not the Lyme, it's something else.

When I was seeing Dr. C and I had the IV PICC line in for a short period, I told Dr. C I needed to be placed on an oral antibiotic. He said, "No, I've cured you!" Three weeks later, I was flat on my back again, unable to move. Had I not gone too see Dr. J when I did, I fear I would have been either in a wheelchair or would have died back then. So, as far as I'm concerned, he saved my life!

But it scares me to death and I know that other chronic Lyme patients feel this way; we are so afraid that the insurance companies and the Conduct Boards may try to intervene with our doctors who treat us. We need our doctors; many others are suffering needlessly at the hands of the insurance companies who want to call the shots.

We need to outline adequate care for Lyme by receiving a proper diagnosis, reliable tests, and making sure that we are covered by insurance companies. I believe that the insurance companies are the ones who are predicting what and who a doctor can treat and what he can't. While we Lyme disease patients remain ill, we suffer at the hands of the insurance carriers.

There have been doctors who treat long-term chronic patients, who have lost their license, who have lost their homes, their families, and some have even committed suicide. We also need to establish research on finding a cure for chronic Lyme disease. The physicians and the media need to be educated on what the tell-tale signs and symptoms a patient may have to detect Lyme disease, proper testing methods, and preventative methods to avoid getting this.

More research and funds need to be allocated so that we Lyme disease patients and families can get at the root of the problem that causes this disease, rather than treating the symptoms.

This disease is heart wrenching and very disturbing. I know of Lyme patients who have no one to turn to; their families ignore their help, they won't speak to them, their doctor's ignore their pleas, insurance companies won't help them either. I have a friend in Michigan who has chronic Lyme disease and my heart just aches for him when I call him on the phone. I wish I had extra money in the bank just so I could go pick him up and take him to Dr. J for treatment. He can barely speak, he stutters terribly, he has Bell's Palsy, he can't remember who he's talking to, or what he's talking about. I sympathize with him because I have gone through the stuttering, memory lapses in and out, and I know how difficult it is and how this makes him feel. I have been blessed with a wonderful, understanding husband and a loving family who have encouraged me to fight for my life, which I have done and continue to do on a daily basis. Unlike my friend in Michigan, his wife left him, his son won't speak to him, his daughter never calls him, he lost his job, his car, and his house. He lives in a rented room in a rundown neighborhood and he's lost the most precious gift—his dignity and self-respect!

I try to encourage him and give him hope that he will get through this, but he can't afford to get an antibiotic to help alleviate his symptoms. There were times when I called him and I would hold my breath for fear that he committed suicide, because of the time it took for him to reach the telephone. I would say, "Where were you?"

He'd reply, "I couldn't get to the phone because I was so tired and sick from trying to get off my chair."

"Thank God, you're all right!" I've never met this man, but I know he's hurting and it hurts me that he is being denied proper care.

At the present time, I am off the antibiotic and using all natural alternatives to see if my immune system can function on its own. Yes, I know antibiotics are not the safest drug to be using but, we have no alternative, this is all we have to try. There's no test to determine if we are in remission.

I've been in the emergency room several times with severe symptoms, fevers, chest pains, numbness in arms and legs, vomiting out of control, and the shakes. Then the emergency room doctors put me through all the grueling tests, blood work, EKG's, X-rays, MRI's, oxygen sensors, and everything comes back normal. The doctor comes into the room, and we can't find anything wrong, so my husband proceeds to tell them, "My wife has Lyme disease."

Their response is, "I don't know what to do for her, obviously you know more about this disease than we do."

I remember a time when I was in hospital #2, waiting for my medical doctor to stop in to see how I was doing. I had numerous thoughts rambling through my mind, like "What will my diagnosis be this time?" In fact, while I was in that particular hospital, the medical staff sent in a priest to pray for me, which I refused to have him do. I kindly asked him to leave me alone and he did, no questions asked. So, while I was lying there in my bed waiting for my lunch tray to arrive, I was actually starting to get an appetite. When this stately doctor in his suit, tie, and white coat appeared at my doorway, I didn't recognize him. You have to understand, I had just so many doctors coming and going that day I couldn't be sure. I asked him, "Who are you?"

"I'm Dr. K."

"Okay, what kind of doctor are you?"

He replied, "I'm a Psychiatrist!"

I thought for a moment, and I may have even started to cry. So this is what they think, that I'm crazy now!

Dr. K said, "I thought we could discuss your anxieties."

"Anxieties" What are you talking about? I'm not depressed or a manic depressed woman." Luckily for him, I could hear the food cart arriving at my room and I was hungry and angry. On my food tray I had a bowl of vegetable soup, a sandwich, and a bowl of Jell-O. I was thrilled to finally get to eat something. Then Dr. K said, "Let's talk."

I was so disgusted with the sight of him that I picked up my food tray and threw at him! He just stood there. I don't think he was too happy with me at that point, but I didn't care what he thought.

In the meantime, while I have been searching and trying to figure it all out, I had several doctors tell me that maybe you need to get some supplemental help, social security, or whatever. I felt degraded over that comment and ashamed.

I started asking around, checking with lawyers that understood Lyme disease to help me get some assistance. Lyme disease lawyers are few and far in between. This would be a task to find one.

In 1999, I filed a disability claim to receive Social Security benefits. What a three- ring circus this turned into. I had heard how easy it was to get it; I mean, people with depression or people who are obese can get it quickly, why can't I, I thought? I was told by the Social Security Administration (SSA) they have their own set of rules as to who gets what or whether you are sick enough or disabled enough to receive help.

I was unable to hold a job because I am too sick to work or perform tasks, even to this day. I've often thought of returning to work, but I know I wouldn't hold out long.

Then I had to go clear back to 1995 when I started having all of these difficulties with my health. The SSA sent me to numerous doctors to do performance tests and see if I was capable of working again. They did a history on me of Present Illness, Review of Symptoms, Allergies, Medications, Illnesses, Injuries, Surgeries, Hospitalizations, and a Family History. Then the physical exams began: Vital Signs, Temperatures, Pulse Rates, Respiration, BP, Mental Status, Psychiatric Evaluations, Eyes, Ears, Nose, Throat, Neck, Lungs, Heart, Abdomen, Back, Lower Extremities, Skin, Neurological, Laboratory-Blood Work, X-Rays, EKG's, Liver Function Tests, Cardiac, and Upper GI. You name it, they ran it!

I went through this for four years. I finally found a lawyer in Cleveland, Ohio, who from another patient gave me their name. I called and scheduled an appointment and met the attorney. My youngest daughter, Corinne, drove me up and we met with my attorney. The attorney told me, "Janet, there are 9,000 cases (me included) and 13 judges to hear cases. This could take up to another 4 years before it comes up in front of a judge."

Before we see a judge, we may be looking at the year 2003. If, for some unforeseen reason he doesn't see you, you could file a Discrimination Suit against them, but not now.

My attorney was in touch with my Lyme disease doctor. The doctor gave my attorney my capabilities and limitations. My attorney has won seven Lyme disease cases so far. My attorney also stated, "You haven't worked for three years, you would think that the SSA would realize you're incapable and unable to hold a job, but they don't." Because my attorney also told me that if you're psychological or obese, you can instantly get it. That's not fair!

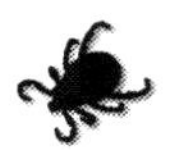

Psychological:

HOW TO DEAL WITH LYME DISEASE

In 1999 I had a difficult time with my speech patterns; I slurred, my husband and family would become agitated with me and would even laugh at me. I guess I sounded like the town drunk. I had memory lapses, I would drive to places, stores, etc., where I'd been countless times but could not remember how to get home. When I was in the grocery store, my grocery cart would be full and I would start to panic and wonder why I was there. Many times, I left my grocery cart loaded in the store and returned home. When I arrived home, I wondered where my groceries were.

I would park my car in the store lot and then couldn't remember where I parked it. When I did locate my car, I would get in and sit and cry because then I couldn't remember how to get home. There were times when I would need to ask or call for directions to get home. I experienced occasions of talking to someone and totally forgot who or what I was talking about. "What did I just tell you?" I'd ask. Some would respond, some laughed, some made shrill remarks, and some were understanding. I wouldn't go outside to visit other family members and friends or even call them. I would rather stay home in my surroundings; it was easier this way, no one could hurt me or make nasty comments to my face. I had a great deal of difficulty with walking, I had no balance and it wasn't pretty to watch. It was difficult to want to join in on fun activities or just to go out to dinner with others for fear I might stumble around or talk like "Porky Pig." Many times while I was making a pot of tea on the stove I forgot the stove was left on. I live 400 feet off the road and I would wobble down to get the mail; I'm sure I was quite a sight to watch as I stumbled around. There were many onlookers who went to great distances to watch me; many times I wanted to "flip them off," but I didn't. What are you staring at you moron! I often took my cell phone with me in case I couldn't make it back to the house. There was a day when that happened; I walked down to the mailbox, I was exhausted, and my chest hurt severely. I called my neighbor and she drove down, picked me up, and drove me up to the house. She wanted me to call my husband, I think she thought I was having a heart attack, but I made her swear on a bible not to tell him. Her husband and my husband are good friends. This was my way of protecting him; he had been through so much with me that I wouldn't and couldn't tell him. I rarely discussed how I was feeling with him, but he already knew just by my body language and could tell that I wasn't feeling well. After all, we've been married for thirty-three years and he knows me like a book!

I have been journaling ever since I developed Lyme disease. My youngest daughter, Corinne, gave me a journal for my birthday, and I write in this book every day. My Lyme disease doctor, Dr. J, also encouraged me to write on everyday experiences and frustrations. "You will have many," he once told me. It has encouraged me to do many feats of which some I'm proud and some I'm not. But the most amazing thing that I have discovered from having this disease is leaning on Jesus. Many a day and night, I would pray to him for strength, help, and mercy to get me through yet another day. And he has done that! Twelve years later, I am still among the living; I'm still here, and I lean on his love constantly.

I have discussed this with many other Lyme patients who have become my friends that I'm grateful I have Lyme disease. Now I don't take life for granted, and no matter how painful this ordeal is or how sick I have been, I am not going to quit; I'm not out of the woods yet but I will trust Jesus with my life.

Experts say tick-borne diseases are often overlooked, misdiagnosed, and never addressed. Veterinary scientists say disease-carrying ticks are migrating like never before, with populations bolstered by warmer temperatures, the rising deer populations, and reforestation. The problem is, the medical community doesn't have the proper testing, knowledge, and education that vets have on tick-borne diseases. Veterinary medicine and human medicine need to work closer to understand tick-borne illnesses.

FOUR MAIN TICKS PLAGUE ANIMAL AND HUMAN MEDICINE

1. Lone Star Tick Carries Ehrlichia Chaffensis, this is the most common form of human ehrlichliosis in the U.S.
2. The Black-Legged or Deer Tick Carries Lyme disease
3. The American Dog Tick Carries primary vector of Rocky Mt. Spotted Fever
4. The Brown Dog Tick Carries Babesia, Ehrlichia canis, but actually is not a vector to humans in North America

Deer are primary reproductive host for black-legged and lone star ticks and are closing in on neighboring suburbanites. So many of us enjoy our half-acre lots, but it can also put us in harm's way. Any given night a raccoon can run onto your property, a tick can drop off, lay eggs, and start a cycle in your backyard. This has been going on for thousands of years. What we need to talk about is our changing relationship with nature. With hunting restrictions for deer, the deer population is growing. There again, we are in harm's way. Dogs *do not* transmit tick-borne diseases—a fact that needs to be understood.

The more ticks there are, the more diseases will emerge. Because the white-tailed deer is the main carrier of Lyme disease, if we don't curtail the population, it's going to become an epidemic of health-related problems.

I've lived on farmland all of my life. I wouldn't change a thing about living out in the country. I never actually gave it a thought. I would lie outside in the grass with my girls at night and look up at the stars, walk through the woods with my girls and our dogs, and collect wildflowers in those high prairie grasses and weeds.

Now, I'm more cautious! We have numerous deer that roam all over our property; they visit our pond for drinking water, eat acorns under the tree, and sometimes they eat my flowers and my ornamental bushes in my landscaping. I check my little pug, Lotus Blossom, when we walk around by those areas for ticks on her skin. Even when my granddaughter, Monet, comes over, I don't allow her to lie on the grass under the tree for fear she may end up with a nasty tick.

We can respect our beautiful world but be very cautious with it. There are life forms lurking out there, and it's not worth the risk that might make you its next victim.

Adult ticks are most active during the fall months. There is data that has been compiled stating forty-eight states have already tested positive this year for Lyme disease exposure. That should be a warning signal for families and your pets.

Why is Lyme disease on the rise? One theory is from global warming; we have warmer temperatures, increased white tailed deer populations, and urban land developers. We need diagnostic screening for our veterinarians so they can properly indentify these vectors. As the tick population continues to grow and migrate, new diseases are introduced and ticks become more likely to carry and transmit a host of diseases. Unfortunately, I became a host for the ticks, and now I'm trying my best to help prevent you from going through what I've had to live with for the past twelve years.

It's extremely important for you to inspect your dogs or cats after they have been outside. When you stop and think about the likelihood of this happening to you, it's terrifying, but it doesn't have to be. Let common sense prevail and use caution! Most pet owners have become more dependent on their furry friends; they play outside, they come inside, they ride in our cars, they lay on our furniture, and many even share your bed with you. Does it ever cross your mind what your furry friend may have lurking on his or her skin? I never gave this a second thought, but I do now!

It's a shame how we take our livelihood for granted; I never thought how dangerous just going for a walk in the woods could be. It's very important to take your furry friends to veterinarians so they can be checked year round for heartworms, flea, and tick prevention. Dog owners shouldn't panic; we should use steps in keeping our pets from wandering around areas that may be attractive to them. Pet owners can visit www.dogs&ticks.com to learn more about ticks and prevention.

Methods of controlling ticks in wildlife parks have been used for the white-tailed deer. It's a contraption or a feeder that the deer walk through; it coats their skin with a repellent against ticks. Any rodent can also carry this vector-borne disease from the white-tailed deer. Even a migrating bird or a white footed mouse, raccoons, and squirrels can be a host and carry this tiny little insect into your backyard.

Deer hunters are another concern to me. I have written articles to a local hunting newspaper warning hunters to be careful.

This article was in the Fish & Field Report on November 1, 2000, Anti-Tick Tips:

HOW TO STAY SAFE FROM LYME DISEASE

Deet is an active ingredient in mosquito repellents. There are pros and cons to each product, but they say as a tick repellent, permethrin wins hands down. Permethrin is an insecticide derived from a chemical found in the chrysanthemum family of plants. It is a spray that is used on clothes only and is deactivated by the oils on your skin. Once it is sprayed on our clothing, it becomes odorless and can last several weeks with a single application. Once it is applied, most ticks will curl up and fall off if they make contact, in which case they will eventually die if there is prolonged exposure.

As I said before, there are pros and cons. Deet has been associated with human case histories of neurological damage and even death. Permithrin has been implicated in possibly contributing to the Gulf War Syndrome. I chose not to use chemicals on myself because of the dangers and allergic reactions I have already developed from having chronic Lyme disease.

I never gave Lyme disease a thought because I'd never heard of it. It's truly amazing how educated and aware you become when you've been stricken with a disease like this.

Who would have ever thought that this tiny insect could cause such an array of symptoms? Lyme disease is the second-fastest growing infectious disease, with only AIDS ranking higher. Of course, you are at a higher risk for this disease if you live in the Northeast, upper Midwest, or Pacific Northwest regions, where deer ticks are more prevalent.

These little bloodsuckers commonly thrive in wooded area with dense brush and shrubbery and are more likely to arise in the spring and fall months[5].

But please don't let ticks terminate your outdoor activities. Just take precautions, be wise, and possibly you can outsmart these critters from making you their next meal and keep you safe from Lyme disease.

I tell landscapers that I've met on the dangers of this disease, and one of the landscapers that works around my doctor's office has talked to me about ticks. He said, "Janet, I've watched you come into this office for five years, and I don't want to end up like you are. I've seen you at your worst days and now your good days, and I am very cautious." But really, any occupation that extends to working outside should be made aware of the dangers. This is nothing to mess with; it has debilitating affects on one's livelihood.

Ticks have been a nuisance since the beginning of time; they pose a danger to humans, to pets, and the wildlife that carry them. I'm very afraid that the U.S. and surrounding countries are going to explode with Lyme disease cases. There has been data by the veterinary industry showing that dogs in forty-eight states already have tested positive for Lyme disease exposure. As the tick populations continue to migrate, new diseases are being introduced at an alarming rate, which can result in a multitude of diseases.

When I was first diagnosed with Lyme disease, I was unprepared for what I was about to experience. I wasn't able to leave my home; I was too weak. My husband had to help me get out of bed so I'd be downstairs for the visiting nurses to come and set up the IV pole along with the mobile X-ray technician.

The nurse would sometimes have to stick me with the needle several times in order to get my vein to pop up so they could guide the PICC line in. Many times when the nurse would do this, blood would squirt out onto the floor. What a mess! My girls, Carrie, who was nineteen, and Corinne, who was sixteen, would usually be there, and my sisters would come over to watch this procedure being performed. Even then, I felt like a bug under a microscope with people poking and prodding at me.

I blamed God for this happening to me and I was angry, very angry. Why was this happening to me? What on earth did I do to deserve this? Why can't someone who's violent or bad have this? Then I would ask the nurses, "How long am I going to have to go through this?"

She stated, "It takes about four to eight weeks, every day, for a short treatment."

I said, "You're kidding, right? Everyday for that long? Am I going to get better? Will I be able to move around on my own? Will I live through all of this?"

All they would say was, "It takes time and depends on the patient." It has been one obstacle after another in those twelve years, I have recovered somewhat, but I have a long way to go yet. I'm learning how to cope with this disease.

Yes, I went through some major depression. I just wanted to lie down and die! Many days I felt so frustrated, guilty, hateful, and I had a great deal of self-pity. The nurses, my sisters, and my family, all tried to encourage me, and I would just sit and stare out the window watching life pass me by. I couldn't think. I couldn't walk without assistance, I couldn't hear or feel; my mind was so muddled with confusion; the drugs I was taking kept me pretty confused and I felt adrift.

One day, I overheard a friend of mine ask the nurse, "How long is she going to have this disease?" The nurse replied, "Until this disease takes her life! It could be soon—months or years—but she's not going to be cured of it, it will only progress!" That made me sick to hear that! How dare they talk about my outcome with this disease? Who did she think she is? I wished they would all go away and just leave me alone.

I had terrible mood swings, I wasn't able to laugh or make jokes, and I didn't like it when anyone else would either! My husband was so down at times with me, I know it had to be heart wrenching for him to see his wife like this. I know he was concerned about our health insurance and bills, and the weight was bearing down on him. I also think he was scared to death that I would die and leave him.

We purchased an RV motor home so we could take our daughters on camping trips and vacations. Our initial plan was that I would return to work and help him pay for this. Well, that plan went south. We ended up selling the RV and had to tighten our belts. Now the ball was in my husband's court; he was a lone survivor having to carry all the responsibilities himself. I felt horrible and responsible for this happening to him. I was a rock tied around my husband's neck and I know he felt like it too, but he never said.

I refused help. My older sisters would send me encouraging cards and pray for me. This only made me angrier, and the more they tried, the angrier I became and the more hateful I was! I would tell them, "Don't talk to me about your God, how loving he is, because I don't care!" This went on for several months and even years. I didn't want to accept any responsibility for myself, my actions, or my feelings. As time went on with this disease, my heart, my feelings, and my attitude started to take on a new meaning.

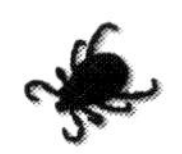

Living with Lyme:

HOW MY LIFE HAS CHANGED

I was finally realizing that having Lyme disease was not my fault. I was learning to lean on God to help me deal with it all. With the help of my sister-in-law (who's more like a sister), who also suffers with a deadly disease, I realized that you have to reach out to people and let them help you. I knew I would be in for a long haul but I wasn't going to give up the fight, no matter what!

My oldest sister, Marg, was more like my mother; there was quite a difference in our ages; she was in her sixties and me in my forties. I spent many summer days with her and her children. She was very faithful to her God; a wonderful, caring woman, fun to be with, a hard worker, a great cook, and she would tell me stories of her childhood.

When she became ill with colon cancer, I was always trying to make her laugh. I'd send her funny stories from the Internet, ornery jokes, anything I could think of to help ease her pain and keep her going.

When she learned of my diagnosis with Lyme disease, she was there for me. She lifted my spirits and helped me to realize how precious life was and not to be afraid of telling God our problems. I fought her tooth and nail when it came to God. I didn't want to hear about him. But as time went on, I watched my sister struggling with her pain and saw how strong her faith was. I began to question. "Who is this God she believes in? And if God is so loving, why does she have to suffer for such a long time? If God really loves her, why does she have to endure all this pain?"

Many times when she was lying in bed she would tell me that there were angels all around her, and I would just sit and look at her, not understanding what she was telling me. Then my sister sent me a card one day saying, "Just to let you know that you are in my prayers. It's such a bummer to be down, but we know it's for a reason. Rest and look to Jesus. He knows our suffering. Be a good patient, now! Love, Marg."

From that time forward I finally understood what she had been trying to tell me about God's love and about being faithful to him. Instead of me being stubborn and relying on myself, I slowly understood everything Marg had taught me about God's love and God healing us in his time.

I finally let God into my heart, and I began to change; life seemed a bit easier, and I knew I would be in for a long battle. I had a lot of negativity inside and felt like I was worth nothing, no self-confidence, impatient, mean, and hateful. If there's anything at all that I've learned about how to deal with a chronic illness is you have to have a positive outlook. It took a while, but once I got over my self-pity, stubbornness, and dependency on drugs to make me feel better.

I had to learn how to find self-worth again, to relearn to be happy, and have self-control again. It was a difficult journey, to say the least, and I knew I was headed for an uphill battle. I have found that you can look at living with a chronic illness in two ways: You can either be happy, learn, or accept what it is that you have and find ways to cope with the illness to make your life more bearable, or you can be mean, spiteful, and hate the world around you, which makes the illness harder to live and cope with.

I have chosen to accept it, find ways to live with it, find physicians to help me cope with this illness, and get on with life. Some of my Lyme friends are really struggling with this disease and are bitter because of it, and some are trying their best. It's extremely frustrating; it has been an ordeal for me and for thousands of others. Of course, it's good to have a positive support team, and I did for a long time. But that has withered away, especially with some of my family members. People do not really know the impact of how this disease has affected me and how it has infected my mind, body, and soul. I've had this for such a long time and, on top of it, I have developed other health problems along the way.

One of my dearest friends also suffers with this disease; she can't get a positive reading for the Lyme. I feel her frustration because she has all the clinical symptoms of it. But this is not unusual; many Lyme disease patients have never been able to get a positive reading. Lyme disease is also known as Lyme Arthritis, Lyme Encephalopathy, Lyme Meningitis, Lyme Borreliosis, Tick-Borne Borreliosis, Neuroborreliosis, and Borreliosis[6].

If a patient is currently on, or has recently taken, antibiotics, the antibacterial effect of antibiotics can reduce the body's production of antibodies. If the patient has or is currently taking anti-inflammatory steroidal drugs (such as those taken to treat rheumatoid arthritis) or certain cancer drugs, these can suppress a person's immune system, thus reducing or preventing an antibody response.

I figured when I would turn sixty or so I would be faced with some kind of illness. In my family history, cancer and heart disease runs pretty thick. But in 1995 I had a tick bite that has changed my life drastically.

PREVENTING TICKS

1. Avoid tick-infested areas, such as dense, wooded areas, tall grasses, woodpiles, especially in May, June, and July.
2. Wear long pants tucked inside of your socks or boots and a long-sleeved shirt tucked inside your pants.
3. Wear white or lightly colored clothes, so you can easily spot ticks.
4. Use an insect repellant that contains Deet on your clothing, sparingly and with caution.
5. Keep areas around your home and garden clear of leaves, brush, and tall grass by keeping your grass cut short.
6. Remove vegetation close to your home that may attract deer and put up barriers to discourage deer from coming close to your house.
7. Place bird feeders away from your house to keep ticks they carry at bay.

8. If ticks are a problem on your property, you may consider having tick pesticides applied to your yard and surrounding areas.
9. If you are in a highly infected tick region, inspect yourself carefully and remove any ticks.
10. After you've been outdoors, check yourself from head to toe, behind your ears, hairline, underarms, under your breasts, and between your thighs. They go where it's warm and moist, just beware!
11. If a tick bites you, save the tick and bring it to your doctor for analysis to determine if it may be a carrier of Lyme disease.
12. If you think you may have Lyme disease, look for telltale signs and see your doctor fast.

SYMPTOMS OF LYME DISEASE

- ☐ Rash—at site of bite/on other parts of the body—circular, spreads out
- ☐ Raised Rash—disappears and reappears
- ☐ Unexplained hair loss
- ☐ Headache, mild or severe seizures/pressure in head, white matter, lesions on head
- ☐ twitching of facial or other muscles/facial paralysis
- ☐ Tingling of nose, tip of tongue, cheek or facial flushing
- ☐ stiff neck and jaw

- ☐ unexplained dental problems
- ☐ sore throat, clearing throat, phlegm, hoarseness
- ☐ pain or swelling in or around eyes
- ☐ increased floating spots/oversensitivity to light
- ☐ buzzing, ringing, or pain in ears/oversensitivity to sounds
- ☐ digestive, excretory systems, diarrhea, constipation, irritable bladder or interstitial cystitis, upset stomach
- ☐ bone pain, joint, pain or swelling, carpal tunnel, stiffness of joints, back, neck, tennis elbow
- ☐ muscle pain or cramps (Fibromyalgia)
- ☐ respiratory and circulatory systems
- ☐ chest pain or rib soreness
- ☐ night sweats or chills
- ☐ heart blockage
- ☐ neurologic system
- ☐ burning or stabbing sensations in the body
- ☐ fatigue, chronic fatigue syndrome, weakness, peripheral
- ☐ poor balance, dizziness, difficulty walking, lightheadedness, wooziness
- ☐ increased motion sickness
- ☐ mood swings, irritability, bipolar disorder, depression
- ☐ disorientation (getting or feeling lost)
- ☐ feeling as if you are losing your mind/panic attacks or anxiety
- ☐ over-emotional reactions, crying easily

- ☐ too much sleep or insomnia/difficult falling or staying asleep/narcolepsy, sleep apnea
- ☐ lost mental capability/confusion/difficulty thinking
- ☐ difficulty with concentration or reading
- ☐ speech difficulty (Slurred/slow/stammered)
- ☐ forgetting how to perform simple tasks
- ☐ sexual dysfunction/loss of sex drive
- ☐ menstrual pain/irregularity
- ☐ breast pain/discharge
- ☐ testicular or pelvic pain
- ☐ unexplained weight gain or loss
- ☐ extreme fatigue
- ☐ swollen glands/lymph nodes
- ☐ fever (high or low grade)
- ☐ continual infections: Urinary Infections, Bladder Infections, Yeast Infections, Ear Infections, Kidney Infections, Eye Infections, Throat Infections, Lung Infections
- ☐ symptoms come and go/pain migrates (moves to different parts of the body)
- ☐ low body temperature
- ☐ allergies and chemical sensitiveness
- ☐ increased effect from alcohol [7]

It's complicated when you have this disease; there's a multitude of symptoms that we deal with. Lyme disease mimics many other diseases such as: MS, MD, Lupus, Chronic Fatigue, Fibromyalgia, Rheumatoid Arthritis, IBS, Allergies, Cerebral Palsy, Lou Gehrig's Disease, Heart Re-Lated Diseases, Immune System Deficiencies and yes, even cancer. It's a myriad of all these diseases rolled into one neat little package, the Spirochete bacterium, known as Lyme disease.

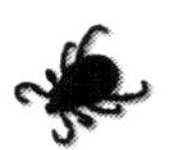

Controversies with Lyme disease:

THE LYME STIGMA

Our biggest problem right now as of 2008 is the IDSA (Infectious Disease Society of America). They are not relying on science of the disease, and they are more interested in relying on their opinions than fixing the problem.

The guidelines for Lyme disease are so strict and controversial, it seems as though the IDSA (Infectious disease society of America) limit certain types of diagnoses, and if the Lyme patient doesn't show or have proof of having the disease, they won't get any treatment or the treatments they have been receiving are dismissed!

The national guidelines issued by the IDSA recommend that doctors give patients with Lyme disease ten to twenty-eight days of an oral antibiotic, with another month allowed for persistent symptoms. But the guidelines now posted on the website for IDSA deny the existence of "Chronic Lyme disease," saying there's no medical evidence that the bacterium causes Lyme. They have also emphasized that a patient has to have the classic bull's eye rash or blood tests to determine a diagnosis of this disease.

Many Lyme disease patients had the bull's eye rash but, because of our "mainstream medical community" and the labs that didn't recognize what it is or even test for it, they fall by the wayside. To top it off, these tests for Lyme disease are not reliable; there are many false negative results.

Many physicians have had to go on symptoms instead of accurate blood readings because of the unreliability of testing procedures performed. For many, the traditional course of antibiotics has worked. I know many patients who were on antibiotics for four years or more, and they are doing fine now. Then there are others who are not fairing as well.

The sad part of all of this is the prestige the IDSA carries and how the insurance companies are beginning to react toward some Lyme disease patients; they may refuse covering them. This will also pose a problem with the new guidelines from IDSA who could stifle new treatments, because doctors will fear they will be disciplined if they step out of the guidelines.

Our pharmaceutical companies make a huge amount of money off Americans, and our health hasn't improved. It's people like myself, my husband, and other Lyme disease activists who are taking a stand for what's right to get Lyme disease into the forefront in the papers, on TV, and rally for support so we can be respected and live with dignity and not be ashamed for having Lyme disease.

It makes me sick when people say, "Oh Lyme disease, that's all?" I wouldn't wish this on my enemies, if I had any. Another comment we get from others include, "You don't look sick." A friend who has this disease for a very long time says she gets that thrown in her face, and it really hurts.

Lyme disease can be a very debilitating disease but, as I've learned by using traditional medicine, the antibiotics can work alongside the natural medicines. Now, if we could just get our "mainstream medical community" to work alongside our naturopathic physicians, we'd have something.

Insurance companies do not want to cover Lyme disease because it can take a long time to get the disease under control, if at all. There's a growing fear that Lyme disease patients won't be able to get their antibiotics because of the guidelines being posted. It is terrifying to think that you need a certain prescription to make you feel better, you are very sick, and you can't get it. Is this a way of "mass reduction" in people; we can't get our prescriptions, so we are just supposed to give up and die?

Many of us struggle with taking the outcome of our healthcare into our own hands. Then we have to come to the realization that this horrible disease may cause feelings of debilitation; this disease can change your life and change your family's stability beyond belief. There's a huge possibility you are not going to make it, you will become disabled, you will have the heartache of being alone and stranded, and then you will die and no one really cares or can help you.

This is why so many Lyme disease patients become an authority on their disease; we have been pushed around and ignored, and we are sick and tired of this treatment. Yes, you do become very educated while you have this disease. We have to stay alert and research, study, and figure out what our next move is. This is like playing a game of chess—good doctors versus bad doctors, good medicine versus bad medicine. It's not been an easy ordeal; not only does the Lyme patient suffer, but the spouses and family are hurt by all of this. To have to watch a human being go back and forth from doctor to doctor with no answers is as frustrating to them as it is to the patient. I'm *Ticked Off.* I say I have had Lyme disease and Rocky Mt. Spotted Fever for twelve years, but being that there is no reliable tests to determine for certain I may have had it longer; who knows!

I never dreamed I'd end up with this. This is a nightmare that never goes away. It's hard to explain to others who do not understand what this is like to live with. I was always pretty healthy, so this was a blow to me. I can't do the activities I once enjoyed. It has changed me drastically; I'm not even sure who I am anymore. Even the shape of my body has changed drastically. I've never weighed this much, and my body doesn't move like it did before I became ill. It is a heartache; life is just revolving around me and I can't be a part of it like I was before.

I have a difficult time working outside in the yard for long periods of time. At one point in my life I raised a huge garden and preserved all the delicious delicacies that I grew. The gardens are all grown over with weeds and brush. We have a huge yard, a pond, a barnyard, and a model field for small, radio-controlled airplanes (which we no longer have.) Once upon a time, I mowed all of it, and I even trimmed the place. Not anymore! I have a beautiful home, raised two beautiful girls, and have a special husband who has been a supportive and loving man throughout it all. But even now my home is a trap for me because I can't take care of it properly.

My daughters helped as much as they could, but with Corinne living in New York City now, she has her own life and job responsibilities. Carrie has her new home; she's a working mom, has a husband, Troy, and daughter, Monet. She has her responsibilities too. I don't expect my husband, David, to help me around the house, but he does when he can. He has enough on his plate with keeping everything mowed, trimmed, and trying to pay the bills and keep his business running.

"Destructive" is putting it mildly when you suffer with Lyme disease, it can be devastating. If you don't stay on an antibiotic long enough, this nasty little creature can pull a protective shell, or cyst, around itself only to emerge later. Isn't that a pleasant thought? You may have a creature inside your body; God only knows the damage it is causing. Believe me, I don't concentrate on this thought or else it would drive me nuts. I have chosen to direct and turn my thoughts over to a much higher power.

The use of cortisteroids will replicate the spirochetes—the bacteria that causes Lyme disease. Therefore, you must not have doctors administer steroids to you; you need to avoid them![8]

Knowledgeable doctors who know how to treat Lyme disease believe that steroids can make Lyme chronic. But by the ignorance of the mainstream medical community, the doctors prescribed steroids to control inflammation, with destructive results for their patients.

For the first four years, I had steroid injections for allergies, inflammation, back and joint pain, and sinuses. But now I am cautious, and most of the wonderful doctors that I have now understand and do not prescribe them.

In researching on the Internet I came across a site: www. Clinical TrialStudies.gov[9]. It's a randomized, double-blind, placebo controlled study on Chronic Lyme disease. There are studies being conducted on chronic Lyme disease. But what I would like to see is a clinical trial study using not an antibiotic but some other form of drug. The mainstream medical community and IDSA are complaining about the use of antibiotics and how they can induce super infections from overuse. Well, then, I suggest we try something else. Who knows what a different drug could do for Chronic Lyme disease patients?

I knew of a man in Florida whom doctors treated for Lou Gehrig's disease. For years, he kept telling his wife and doctors he believed he had Lyme disease. But no one in the medical field believed him. So they continued to treat him for Lou Gehrig's disease. He told his wife he wanted to be checked for Lyme disease. The doctors tested him, and he tested positive. But because his body was weakened, it was too late for him to try the IV Rocephrin antibiotic for Lyme disease, and he died shortly after.

Insurance means assurance, and this is another huge impact on Lyme disease patients. I know what I went through with my husband's insurance and how the rates increased. My husband was forced to locate another insurance company for himself so we could afford medical insurance. Every time a doctor would diagnose me with some illness, my rates continued to soar. I knew if I tried to find another insurance company I would be denied, and I was.

I was stuck with this insurance company, and I had to stay on the policy so my medical and prescriptions were covered. The insurance company kept raising my rates; my deductible was already at $1500 per person, and they wanted me off their plan. In the early stage of the disease, the medications were expensive. Just the expense of the IV drip cost the insurance twelve grand. What really caused an issue with my insurance was when Dr. D. told them I had Chronic Fatigue Syndrome; my insurance company went ballistic!

So I went into see Dr. W. for another physical exam in his office on March 3, 1999. He started me with stress management classes, and I managed to work through them. I told Dr. W. that my insurance company was upset about the diagnosis of Chronic Fatigue Syndrome, and they were informing me of the raising of my insurance rates, again. I asked him, "What can you do about this, Dr. W?"

On June 4, 1999, Dr. W diagnosed me again and told me, "Your symptoms that have previously been diagnosed as a Chronic Fatigue Syndrome by your previous physician, Dr. D, have disappeared. With reasonable medical certainty, I feel that you do not have Chronic Fatigue Syndrome and this is more of an anxiety reaction, which you have completed successfully by attending the stress management program."

Dr. W sent a letter to my insurance company to try to get them to understand and not increase my monthly insurance rate. By that time, my insurance was $600 a month, with a $1500 deductible, and a co-pay of $81 for prescriptions.

Just think of the time I lost going from doctor to doctor trying to figure all of this out! There has been a great deal of lost time and money wondering what was wrong with me.

Some doctors are up-to-date on Lyme disease especially Lyme literate doctors whom are very aware of this disease. Many doctors are taught that Lyme disease is rare and easily cured and think that it is not a serious disease.

But it doesn't really come down to the costs or the money, it is the time, the aggravation, and the suffering that has devoured my life and has hurt my husband and my family. There is time that has been lost that I will never get back. All because our mainstream medical community couldn't figure it out. I felt like a deck of cards shuffled from one hand to the next, not knowing what fate was to befall me. That's what has really hurt.

I missed out on all the fun adventures and family time that have been lost in this game of Russian roulette. I feel like I've been stripped, demoralized, and denied my rights of a citizen who—by no fault of my own—ended up with a disease like this.

I suppose at that particular time in my life, I was very bitter. I had a tough time accepting what was happening to me. My family struggled with what I was dealing with, and then they had to watch me go through this as I was slowly being torn apart by the medical profession's abuse. I could see the hurt in their eyes, their voices; how painful to watch a loved one suffer like that!

So I hoped and prayed that my insurance rates would not continue to climb. All I had was hope: hope for strength, hope for happiness, balance, hope that someone, somewhere would reach out to me and give me hope and satisfaction that I can live out my days in dignity for a healthier future, and possibly a cure for this disease.

But then there's a moment when your journey gives you a self-determination, a wonderful self-empowerment that even though you are scared to death at what your outcome may be for the future, you start to take on a new look at yourself, the disease you're fighting, at the ignorance of the mainstream medical community, and know the battle may be long and arduous, but it is slowly becoming your own personal battle.

I am the one who is ill. I have to take a long, hard look at myself, my attitude, my body language, and my faith. But at that time, I had little faith and I feel that made my journey even harder to fight and to live with because of my lack of faith. I could not believe that my life would ever amount to a hill of beans, but boy, was I ever wrong!

Having a disease such as Lyme disease has been a difficult and bumpy road. Maybe if the disease was given the recognition that it deserves, then yes, Lyme disease is a true disease just like all the other diseases. And whether our mainstream medical community and the IDSA want to refute the disease as being "chronic" or not is beside the point. Millions of people in the United States and surrounding countries suffer with this disease and are pushed aside, shoved under the rug, ridiculed, mistreated, and laughed at, but we will not give up, and I will continue to stand up and be heard. I won't back down because I can't afford to do so.

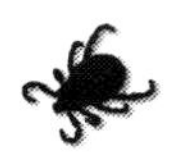

Campaigning For Lyme disease

To raise awareness for Lyme disease, many Lyme patients would go to Washington, D.C., and campaign and walk the halls of justice, speaking to congressional people. The media needs to be made aware and focus on what we are saying; we need to receive the proper help. After all, many would campaign in their own cities and states with high hope and expectations, only to be discouraged. We voice our concerns, our complaints, but they don't hear us!

I came up with the idea to raise awareness in my hometown with the idea aimed at former president George Bush with people all across the country sending in postcards. We told our horror stories in Washington, D.C., during a rally on Capitol Hill.

A dear friend of mine started a support group for the disease. She would march in the rally and then meet with Ohio lawmakers to ask them to support a Congressional Bill asking for $125 million over five years to develop a reliable test, improve tracking, and the reporting of a massive public and doctor education campaign.

Unfortunately, the majority of people who end up with this disease become experts because the mainstream medical community know so little about Lyme disease. My husband and I have researched Lyme and continue to return to the same place of origin, a small island in Connecticut called Plum Island. We feel that Lyme disease is a man-made disease and the Government doesn't want anyone to know about it. The symptoms of Lyme disease were confusing, but our struggles were real, and we were so compelled to help other Lyme disease friends. I wrote an article for our local newspaper, and a cameraman from the paper and a writer came into my home and interviewed me. I felt compelled to let the public know about this mystery disease. It amazes me even to this day and time we still haven't received proper diagnosis; unreliable testing is still a huge factor with this disease, physicians still overlook the signs and symptoms, and we are still trying to get recognition. There are many support groups all over the U.S. and surrounding countries. We are finally developing websites, chat rooms, and we now have research centers who are at least trying to unravel the mysteries of this disease.

I feel it comes down to the money. It's not fair that certain diseases can attract more attention and we can't get Lyme disease the recognition it deserves as well. We finally do have some tests for Lyme disease such as C6 Lyme Peptide, ELISA, and Western Blot. These tests show a sensitive detection of early Lyme disease, a high specificity for Chronic Lyme disease, the differences of positive and negative results. This disease is cognitive, neurological, and psychological as well as physical. If you go undiagnosed for a long period of time, the disease buries itself deeply in your tissues and requires a long treatment with antibiotics and herbal vitamins to help alleviate some of the on-going symptoms.

I know all too well how easy it is to get discouraged. We get tired of the whole scenario, the doctors, the medicines, the vitamins, the lab work, the tests, and the ignorance from our mainstream medical community and the media. We've all been there and still continue to go through this on a daily basis. Some Lyme disease patients just give up; they have lost faith in the system and their doctors who treat them. But I urge you to stick it out, don't quit, keep taking your medications, keep doing whatever it takes to get through the day, the week, the month, and the year.

This is it how it goes, you take the antibiotics, a month goes by, you feel a tiny bit better, but at first you feel awful. Some people think it's the antibiotics, thinking they must be allergic, no rash, no hives, so they quit and go on feeling lousy. But the "lousy" feeling is good. This means the antibiotics are working; they are killing off the spirochetes (the bacteria from the Lyme). They explode inside your body, release toxins, and now your immune system is working overtime. Then the "yuck" goes away, but in four weeks the same thing happens once again. The spirochetes (bacteria from the Lyme) only come into the bloodstream one time a month, and this is when the antibiotics are hard at work. The rest of the time they are hiding in your bones, tissues, and tendons; Lyme disease is a whole body disease and a whole body experience.

My confidence in myself was shattered; I was unsure of who I was and what direction my life was going in. I always enjoyed having family over to visit but even that started to take a toll on my well-being. Just being out around people in general, I was very defensive and fearful, angry, hurt and discouraged. I had no idea what was in store for me. It was just the beginning; I felt like I was traveling down into a long, dark tunnel of no return.

I placed my faith in doctors, and sometimes I think we assume they know everything and act as though they're God, able to help us and heal us. But we know that this is not true, they are just men or women doing a job to the best of their ability, and that's all we can expect of them. If those physicians would have been knowledgeable about diagnosing this disease back then, I wouldn't have experienced the rotating cycle of misinformed doctors who had no clue what was wrong with me.

If you get bit with a tick today and you find a Lyme-literate doctor who knows what tests to issue, they can do amazing treatments to help you recover without any long-term difficulties.

The treatment protocol, however, is antibiotics. It was then and it still is—that's it in a nutshell! We had no choices, and we still don't. In my case, if I stop using the antibiotics, all my symptoms will return in a few short weeks. And you ask me, "How do you know that?" because I have tried stopping the medication. One morning I woke up and said, "I have had enough of this. I'm tired of depending on these medications and vitamin supplements that helped to sustain my life." Well, one week later, I was in trouble; my bones and muscles felt like they were on fire, I felt as though someone poured acid all over me, and my skin just burned. I would become so fatigued just from making my bed that I would lie down and sleep for four hours. Just putting on my shoes exhausted me.

At that time, I didn't know what it meant to be antibiotic free. I needed them. I didn't know how much longer I would be using them. Unfortunately, using the antibiotics was my only weapon in fighting this disease. My biggest concern was building a resistance to the antibiotic. Due to the fact that before I was diagnosed with Lyme in 1999, for those first four years, all those doctors that I'd seen had me on so many different antibiotics, I was sure I would be in trouble with using them. So it goes back to the same question, "What will I do or what will any of us chronic victims use if we can't use the antibiotics?"

Between suffering with the Lyme symptoms and taking the extensive amount of time to treat Lyme disease, coping with it on a daily basis can become a way of life. I have come to what some Lyme disease patients know as a "window in my life". This is the time when the antibiotic treatments were helping, and I could accomplish small tasks that I was usually too ill to deal with. Some of us are fortunate enough in many ways to avoid permanent, physical damage. Had I not been so stubborn and determined to find help when I did by searching the Internet, talking to other Lyme disease victims and finding a Lyme-literate doctor who knew what was wrong with me and having been properly diagnosed, I feel I wouldn't be sitting here today!

I struggled for a long, long time because I was angry with God for letting this happen to me. I had to learn to trust him and then figure it out. While I continued to fight God every step of the way, my struggles with this disease seemed to be even harder to live with. I had many in my family and friends who would pray for me, place me on their prayer chains at their churches, and I was grateful, but I still denied God's love, his help, and grew even angrier with them for trying to comfort me. At the time I didn't know it, but it was God's way of testing me, I guess to see what strengths I had never known I possessed. I tried to do what God wanted me to do, but it was a long, difficult journey.

"Don't talk to me about your loving God and how he loves me. If he loved me, he wouldn't have done this to me." This attitude went on for days, months, and years. I didn't want to accept any responsibilities for myself, my actions, or my feelings. I just wanted it to all end! I've read of many Lyme disease victims who ended their misery. But I couldn't think clearly of a way to do it, and I didn't want to put my family through that. I didn't feel it would be fair to them if I chose to end my life because of the guilt and remorse they would have to live with.

They didn't deserve this and neither did I! And I feared that God wouldn't accept me into his kingdom if I succumbed to committing suicide. That's not the answer, either! So what is the answer? My search of discovering myself in the scheme of things was just beginning. All this started from 1996 to 2000. It was about four years before I finally accepted my illness.

Everyone tried so hard to invite me to church, go see a faith healer, pray, pray, blah, blah, blah, let's go out for lunch and talk. The only thing I wanted to do was just sit and stare out the window. I couldn't think, I couldn't feel, my mind was so muddled with confusion. Most of the drugs I was on had a dire affect on me; I felt like a puppet on a string dancing around to no music. I couldn't walk upright; I was hunched over, pain coursing through my body, nauseous most of the time, sitting in dreadful despair of what was happening to me. I had no control of my life anymore, I had no music in my life, I loved to sing or hum, just be happy, the laughter was gone, the positive outlook missing. I didn't care anymore. I felt as though I was being punished.

I really had a long, long time to think about all of this and the situation I was getting deeper in. I realized with the help of my sister-in-law, who's more of a good friend than a relative, who also suffers with a devastating disease. In fact, at one point in my life

I was jealous of her because she had access to different kinds of medications, trial studies, and clinics that knew how to treat her disease. That's an awful thing to say and to think, but that's how it was! She taught me to re-think my life, to reach out to others and let others help you. Not to give up, but to keep fighting for your life and get out of the pity situation. "We all go through this!" she said.

I was reading a book one afternoon, a true story of death and life by Don Piper called 90 *Minutes In Heaven.* One of the chapters is about endless adjustments, and it made me realize how difficult this journey I'm on living with Lyme disease has been and still is. I am personally going to be in pain for a long time; these are lessons that God puts upon us to shed some light on how we think and feel. I can't refuse help; if someone wants to help me, I need to let them do it.

For years, my husband, David, has wanted me to have someone come into our home and clean for me because I am unable to do it all! It takes me an average of three days to clean the house and about a week and a half to recover. But it was always embarrassing for me to ask for help. Now, twelve years later, I have my niece come in and clean, and it has taken the pressure off me.

I do not know why it is so hard to ask for help. Why do we stress so over this? All I had to do was just ask God for help and guidance. I never understood that concept.

I research constantly, e-mail other Lyme friends, and I've spoken to doctors outside the U.S. and the state of Ohio who are just as bombarded with this disease. I've spoken to doctors in Canada and Switzerland about their treatment protocols, the complexities of Lyme disease, and the loss of patients through experimental treatments. I've picked at their minds, learning as much as possible about Chronic Lyme disease and which antibiotic and other medications are most effective.

In 2001 I received an e-mail about a new Swiss treatment for Lyme disease, so I checked it out. This was just an experimental measure called ICHT (Intracellular Hyperthermia Therapy), where they go into your body and heat your cells from the inside out. This particular Austrian physician successfully treated another spirochete that crosses Syphilis with Malaria to induce high fevers. This approach has not been accepted and there wasn't a success rate for performing this on cancer and Lyme disease patients.

It was also extremely expensive, and most insurance companies do not cover if out of the U.S. To me and my doctor at the time, it sounded inadequate, unpredictable, and possibly dangerous. My doctor also mentioned that it could affect my cardiopulmonary functions, psychological functions, and might damage cells. Now, if it was 100 percent guaranteed to cure Chronic Lyme disease, I'd find the money somehow. To be free of this disease would be amazing![10]

You do need to be cautious when you are Internet searching for cures, and I have read of many people who have gone to great lengths, wasted money, and precious time trying to be alleviated from the pain of this tedious, draining disease. You have to read, ask questions, and be careful while on the Internet because there are scams and people waiting for you to lay your money down, promising you a cure.

One afternoon I picked up the phone and called this particular number to order a vitamin I wanted to try. The number was to a woman who was selling T-shirts. One thing led to another, and I started telling her about Lyme disease when she informed me she also has Lyme disease. Now was this a guardian angel tapping me on my shoulder, telling me to get on with the journey I was supposed to be doing to reach out to others who are hurting? I don't know, but it sure was an interesting day after that.

I care deeply about helping others and have the hunger to learn as much as I am capable to further understand the seriousness of Lyme disease. There is so much work to be done: we need reliable testing, reliable detection, reliable and literate doctors to recognize the symptoms and properly treat the patient without fear of being denied protection from insurance companies, medical conduct boards, and new drugs instead of the old stand-by, the antibiotics. We need clinical trial studies, must educate the public and the media to raise awareness, hold rallies, have walk-a-thons, whatever it takes to get this Lyme disease recognized.

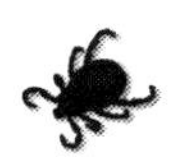

Money and Medical Crusades

A woman traveled to Capitol Hill to lobby for Parkinson's Disease. The hearing rooms upon where she stood were small, the turnout was weak. If she was lucky, she'd get to meet with a representative's legislative assistant, who would only give her ten minutes to talk, but the representative told her, "I'd prefer to wrap this up in five minutes."

When she arrived on Capitol Hill with Michael J. Fox on her arm, those five-minute meetings she tried to conduct turned into one-hour meetings. When Michael J. Fox asked for $75 million in research money for Parkinson's (they managed to get part of it), the hearing room was mobbed and the mood was electrifying.

Now, what's wrong with this picture? It's a cold, mundane, surreal existence of how it really is, of personal tragedies, public promises, and it's sad to report, money, celebrities, and disease have a long tradition of getting what they want![11]

I've read that there's more medical research dollars available than ever before in the National Institute of Health. Diseases without star power struggle for attention. It is unfair that certain diseases attract money just so our politicians can get a signed autograph from them. If this is the way it is, then we need to find a movie star who will help meet our needs. We need public awareness to help raise private funds for medical research.

Maybe it will take someone in the political realm like themselves, their spouses, or children to end up with Lyme disease, and they'll finally see a ray of light. Maybe then the politicians will be more willing to reach into their own deep, dark pockets and help raise awareness.

When my girlfriend and I tried to campaign here at our home for "Have a Heart, Mr. President," all we received was a few horn toots, thumbs up, waves from passersby, and a reporter who didn't do his homework and gave us a bad review.

Many famous people have gotten their share of the pie from the National Institute of Health and politicians to help with funding and research. But there are thousands of Lyme disease support groups around the U.S. who are diligently working on support of Lyme disease bills.

In fact, I have a letter from a former Congressman, addressed to a friend of mine who organized a support group in 2000, thanking her. He was responding to House Bill HR2790, the Lyme disease Initiative. In 1998 alone a total of 15,934 cases of Lyme disease were reported, representing a 24 percent increase since the previous year. He also stated the fact that symptoms of Lyme disease are similar to other illnesses, so diagnosis is difficult. There is not yet a reliable diagnostic test for Chronic Lyme disease. This lack in expertise and knowledge results in prolonged pain and suffering. Each year this disease costs between $1 billion to $2 billion in medical costs.

He was a very sincere congressman who stood by us and kept our concerns in mind. When the House Bill comes to the floor, he told us, "I will consider it." James Traficant-17th District for the State of Ohio, Congressman. The federal government brought him up on racketeering and bribery charges. We feel that he was railroaded into these charges because he spoke his mind! We finally had a ray of hope with a local congressman, and now we have to start all over again looking for a new congressman to stand by us and not against us.[12]

There have been many house bills that have made it to the floor and hopefully there will be many more. We have been trying to raise awareness to designate the month of May as "Ohio Lyme disease Awareness Month" for the sole purpose to raise public awareness of Lyme disease as a health concern.

There was a House Bill 297 Sponsor Testimony given by Rep. Jim Carmichael; the bill has seventeen cosponsors.

I would love to see billboards, trees, and signs posted with green ribbons, displaying public awareness for Lyme disease.

As of 2007–2008, there are many actors, actresses, musicians, writers, and people who are writing books and movies being created on Lyme disease. I just hope we get a deluge of famous people doing whatever they can to raise awareness. We need mass media attention, talk shows with Lyme disease patients, physicians who aren't afraid to speak out about the complexities of this illness and then won't be prejudiced against them for speaking out to raise awareness and help the ones who are in the chronic stages.

I remember when I became deathly ill in the middle of the night, my husband happened to wake up, noticed I wasn't in bed, and came downstairs looking for me. He found me in the kitchen; I wasn't feeling well, I was weak and in pain, and I felt like I was going to pass out. He immediately sat me down on the chair and I could hear him, faintly, calling Corinne to wake up. They both managed to get me to the couch to lie down and called 911. They waited and waited, no siren, no ambulance; I imagined my husband was fit to be tied by that time when our local police officer showed up and wanted to know what was wrong. My husband must have said, "My wife is ill; she needs an ambulance, now!" The police officer was anxious as well as to where the ambulance was.

Finally, Dave and Corinne helped me into our van and started down our driveway, whereupon the ambulance arrived. My husband told them, "You're late. I'm taking her in!" When we arrived at the hospital emergency room I was feeling bad. The nurses were sitting around talking about the parties they went to the night before, the guard was just sitting there at his desk, and I said to my husband, "Honey, I'm not going to make it. I'm sick. I need something to vomit in."

He grabbed the waste can, and I hugged it for dear life and convulsed over and over again in it. Well, they finally started to clean me up and sent me down for tests, blood work, EKG's, IV's, Oxygen, Ultrasounds, X-rays; you name it, I had it! When I finally arrived back into my room, the doctor asked if I'd been ill for long. My husband said "Yes, she has Lyme disease." I guess from what I recall the look on that doctor's face was priceless. As usual, "What's that? I've read about that in my textbooks, but I don't know what to do for her!"

After I vomited five times, I felt wonderful! This reaction I had was caused by a herxheimer reaction. My husband explained this to the ER doctor. "When a person with Lyme disease has an experience like this, you can become extremely ill for days, weeks, and even months. But it's a good thing. When this happens it means that the antibiotic is killing off the bacteria." I signed the release form and came home.When I remember back to those terrifying days and nights of what my family had to experience with me and this disease, I'm befuddled by all of it. The anguish, frustration, emotionally, physically, and mentally, they have experienced with me and the fear they must have felt makes my heart ache. I know that twice when I went into the ER, I didn't know if I'd return home. With all the nurses and doctors swarming around me, poking and prodding at me, I felt like the end was near.

The doctors have told me the longer you have Chronic Lyme disease, the longer it takes to get it under control, if you will be able to at all! Having late-stage Lyme disease can prove to be extremely difficult for some of us. So there are days when it's two steps forward and six steps back; there are setbacks with this.

I have flare-ups with this disease usually about every four weeks and, with a woman, it seems to center around their menstrual cycle. I've suffered with chest pains, fevers, and shakes. I just never knew what I would deal with. And there were times when it might be nothing at all! There were times when my husband would just hold me until the pain subsided. I would use any type of pain reliever over the counter, but nothing seemed to work. So I ended up at my Lyme disease doctor begging him for pain medicine.

He didn't want to prescribe pain medicine, but he also knew the pain would just continue to bombard me and it would only become increasingly worse. So he prescribed Percocet. It was expensive, but I didn't care, I just wanted pain relief. I just wanted relief so I could manage to have some sort of life existence and be without pain on a constant basis. Little did I know I would become very addicted to those little white pills. The Percocet became my little best friends. I ate them like candy; I just wanted to be pain free and sleep.

My husband and daughters were very concerned about this and were not happy with me for using these pills. These pills had a terrifying effect on me and my personality. I couldn't think, I couldn't concentrate, and I was mean! I had a low tolerance that made me get upset easily over the smallest of things. I would sit in silence for many days and months. The most devastating to me as of today is how it's taken my memories away.

There are so many memories I can't remember about my past, my children's childhoods, of what they were like when they were babies, their likes and dislikes, about when they started to walk, and their childhood characteristics. It's just gone; it's as though my mind has been wiped clean. My husband will ask me about when we dated, the things we did, and where we went, and I have no clue what he's talking about. That's tough! I've been married for thirty-four years, and I can't remember important dates or events.

But I am so madly in love with this man, my husband, and even though we've been married that long, he's still standing here beside me, supporting me, laughing with me and loving me while I walk through this journey. Lyme disease affects the mind in a serious way, it's like suffering with a head injury. Lyme disease can often strike at an entire family and the results can be very damaging. It leaves the Lyme disease patient with a higher rate of divorce, family dysfunction, and it has been known to cause domestic violence.

I had a tendency at one time to be obsessive compulsive; when I would leave the house, I'd check my wallet to make sure it was in my purse. My husband would be driving the truck, and I'd be sitting there looking in my purse for my wallet, touching it, opening it up. I had no idea what I was looking for, but I would do this over and over again. Or there were instances when I'd leave the utility room to walk into the garage and turn right back around and make sure the light was off, over and over again. This was probably the worst feeling I had, just being so compulsive about everything. I thought I was going bonkers!

I couldn't multi-task either. I had to do one thing at a time. My poor husband would have to explain over and over again how to do our banking or give me directions. Sometimes I felt like my body was here but my mind was somewhere else—but where? I wrote notes on sticky pads and had them taped all over the kitchen so I could remember what I was doing or what I was supposed to be doing. I know this was all stemming from the side effects of all the medications I was using. I was taking medicine for pain relief, to sleep, antibiotics for the Lyme disease, for anxiety, stomach medicines, plus all the vitamins and supplements I was using on a daily basis. I felt like I had no life, and I really didn't in the beginning.

My husband was trying to keep me interested and involved in his business, to make me feel like a partner with him and to make me feel needed. Even today, I am somewhat involved with the business, but he makes the decisions and I just assist him when needed. It's too stressful, and I don't want the headaches, so I have given back a lot of the responsibilities to him. After all, it's his business, not mine.

Lyme disease produces swelling in the brain; this can affect your ability to process information. This particular location terrifies me because it can affect your thoughts, cause disorientation, lack of concentration, and severe anxiety. I feel I am falling into this category everyday, and it frightens me.

Symptoms can vary and intensify, with stress and fatigue being the major contributors. It's best to avoid, but with life and all its ups and downs, how can it be possible? The disease is compared to riding on a rollercoaster of no return—when will it stop? When will it go?

Who knew that such a tiny insect could cause such havoc in my body and a slow decline of my health? Would I have used more caution when I would go camping or hiking in the woods if I knew what this disease was, and how it would cause such a deadly ordeal to live with? I would have taken precautions and not allowed myself to lie out in the grass or walk around barefoot in my garden.

If Lyme disease was known of and the public was addressed on its dangers, what were the symptoms to look for I would have taken more precautions.

Now, it's the Lyme disease you discuss and the next thing you know you have formed a bond with people. It's amazing how many there are of us with Lyme disease, and we all share that same bond of not knowing what we had for such a long time, due to all the misdiagnosis of our mainstream medical community that they themselves have put upon us. Then I've met many whose disease was caught early; they're all doing fine and enjoying life.

When I first was diagnosed with having Lyme disease in 1999, my husband usually drove me over to Dr. J's office, which was in another state. I had to have someone go into the room with me with the doctor so they could help me to recall my symptoms and to help me to remember directions on taking my medications and so forth. Dr. J. was always very attentive and listened to me. Sometimes it would prove difficult for me to discuss my emotions with him, especially when my husband was present.

I always had a tendency to worry more than I needed, but there were times when I was stressed out from my husband, children and in-laws—they were the problems and the cause of my anguish. The doctor would reassure me that this was normal, that most Lyme patients experienced this and that the family just needs to understand the complexities that Lyme disease brings on a patient. But Dr. J also told my family to keep their comments and frustrations to themselves and not show or direct your emotions toward me. He told them, "This can be very damaging to the patient who has Lyme disease due to the fact that the patient does not need the extra stress!"

When I visited Dr. J, I would also bring all my medications and vitamins along with me so he could determine whether or not I had any reactions to the combinations of drugs and natural products I was consuming at that time. Dr. J was a caring, considerate, and laid-back kind of guy. My husband, the first time he met him, asked questions about the Lyme disease and what to expect and so forth. He really has a great deal of respect for Dr. J, and for everything he did for me. I can't say that about too many physicians that I've seen in twelve years; there are just a small handful of them that I do have a great deal of respect and admiration for.

Dr. J was well informed on Lyme disease and other tick-borne diseases. He was the one who discovered I had Rocky Mt. Spotted Fever from analyzing the spots on my shins. He was the only doctor out of thirteen and three hospitals who had any clue what they were. There is no cure, the medical community does not want to treat the disease due to there's no treatment or cure for it, so their source of revenue dries up (their income) so they don't treat it.

Some doctors will respond to patient input but many do not. If you feel you are not taken seriously, then you need to find a doctor who will listen and learn from you, so you can get the proper treatment. This is why Lyme disease victims educate themselves about Lyme disease and your own doctor may learn as well. *He* and his staff were excellent in their skills and knowledge about these diseases. They gave me a sheet of paper with all the healthy things needed such as rest, exercise, eating the right foods, supplements, and avoiding stress!

He explained the Jarisch-Herxheimer Reaction and what to expect, how easy or severe it could be, depending on the patient. Everyone reacts differently, he would tell us. He told me I would probably have to deal with low blood pressure or high blood pressure, but in my case it registers low. I have it go as low as 110/70, 90/60, 80/50. He also told us that yeast infections can develop. At that time, I was using Diflucan to help alleviate the problem. When you have chronic candidiasis, patients show allergic symptoms to antibiotics. If the patient seems allergic to four or five antibiotics, yeast is probably the problem. Other yeast symptoms are sugar cravings and chronic psoriasis. When you consider all of the antibiotics I was using before I was diagnosed with Lyme disease, you can really understand why I have had such a difficult time using them.

When I had the IV rocephrin drip before I went to see Dr. J in July of 1999. I didn't have the IV on as long as I needed to. Dr. C tried to tell me he cured me, but when I told him that I should be on an oral antibiotic, he refuted. I know some Lyme disease patients who have had a port installed in their chest for replacement of the IV drip, instead of the PICC line through a vein. Not all Lyme disease patients are given IV therapy. After taking an antibiotic for a while, you reach plateaus; sometimes a Lyme disease doctor will incorporate another antibiotic along with it. Then, usually, you can reach a plateau where it becomes effective in your treatment. Of course, it helps to use acidophilus or probiotics while also on the antibiotic.

It was actually easier, mind-wise, to live with the symptoms rather than be ridiculed by the mainstream medical community that I had seen for advice. I lived in constant pain, unable to stand erect without falling over, constant night sweats, insomnia, splitting headaches, strange things happening to my skin (and I still deal with this today.) I feel like an alien is inside me. I felt like yelling and screaming because of what was happening to me.

It seems strange to me that when I went to Dr. J, he wanted to know about my family history and my life. I didn't have any other doctors who wanted to study my life's history like he did. I had seen many specialists, and no one had actually taken a full history on me. At times, I had great difficulty remembering my past, especially when it came to my mother. There were times I blocked out events that had transpired with her that I chose not to remember.

Dr. J wanted me to recall my history: past vacations, present activities, and so on. We told him about having the bull's eye rash on my foot, how Dr. D. treated me for ringworm. I mapped out where it was located on my foot and what it looked like.

After Dr. C finally determined I had Lyme disease, I was relieved. Because now I knew that, after all I'd been through, we finally had some answers. I was degraded by much of the mainstream medical community the labels that they so conveniently marked me with have gnawed at me for many years, mentally, emotionally, and physically, but not spiritually.

Do I feel bitter to those doctors who shamefully put me through this? I did in the beginning, but now I don't. I pity them and pray that by writing this book no one else will fall prey to them. I'm eternally grateful to my Lyme disease doctor, who I feel has saved me from sitting in a wheelchair or even death. I had just seen him in the ample amount of time or else my life could have turned for the worse. I also owe gratitude to many other literate doctors who have and are still doing remarkable things to improve the quality of my life. I know I have benefitted greatly from suffering with Chronic Lyme disease. I've met some remarkable people who tell the same stories of their impossible diagnosis, no one out there to listen to or give them the time of day and to finally reach out and help them. It's been an amazing journey, and I'm still working my way through it.

The majority of the human race has no clue what we go through on a daily basis. I believe I'm growing, and I've become wiser by living with this disease. I have a growing sense of maturity about my illness. I am not so eager to tell anyone what's wrong with me, but I still feel like I'm walking on a thin sheet of ice.

As far as my friendships with other Lyme friends, my sisters and brothers, and friends, I don't go out too often. If I'm planning on an evening out, then I'm required to stay home during the day to rest up for my outing. If I go out during the day by 1:00 p.m. I'm hurting all over and can't wait to return home to sit or lie down. Making commitments for dinner engagements with my husband has subsided considerably. I never was one for going out in the first place, and I thank God that my husband felt the same. The other issue of not going out was my exposure to germs that I may encounter. I can't afford to be around large groups of people, shopping in the malls, eating in restaurants, and being around small children for fear of catching a cold or the flu.

It has been difficult for me to realize how this disease has changed my life but now I know my purpose.

Pain has just become a way of life for me, 365 days, all the time, day and night. It's amazing how a body can endure all this pain for so long. It has taken me a long time to realize how my condition has affected my emotions. The mainstream medical community kept trying to push drugs down me for the pain, for my depression, for the panic attacks. I had so much garbage in my system. I'm surprised I'm still alive! I guess you could say that God has his reasons for why I'm still here: a purpose, a plan, only time will tell.

The best I can say is, don't waste your energy explaining to anyone how you feel; keep focused on your family, who understand what you are dealing with.

Where at one time there was despair and hopelessness, now I feel a renewed sense of hope and pride. My symptoms are improving, but I know I'm far from being over this disease. It is still a journey in the making!

I relish the pastimes I do enjoy, like writing and keeping my journals. I've written poems and prayers that help me release the stress of having and living with a chronic illness.

Oh Lord, fill my heart with laughter and cheer,
To be ever thankful to still be here
To enjoy the wonder that you have created
For all to see and for all to hear.
Your continued love is a reminder of the power
You give to us to use everyday, lest we
Not forget the many things you have done
And will continue to do, if only we Pray. Amen.

Lord, we thank thee for the beauty of this day
And for your glorious message,
Bless this food that's upon this table,
Bless the hands that have prepared it,
Bless those who are not among us
And bless the ones who have gone before us
Restore our faith, our hope and our joy
In Jesus' name, amen.

I wrote a poem about my four-legged furry friend, Lotus Blossom:

There was this little puggy
Who sits upon my lap
She snores like a lion
As she wiggles her fat.
Brown, beige and black
Are the colors of her hair
She hasn't a worry
She hasn't a care

You make me get up and get moving
You like to have fun
But most days you're happy
To just lay around and be a bum.
I love this little puggy
As she sits upon my lap
She snores like a lion
As she wiggles her fat.

I've written many poems and stories and journaled throughout this illness. It is a great inspiration and extremely therapeutic to sit down and write out my thoughts, my struggles, and my pain. The journaling is a place where I can go and explain my feelings without being judged. I have seven of them now, and I continue to write. I have encouraged many others to try to evaluate their lives, hurts, misgivings, and remembrances. Sometimes I find it difficult to lay the pen down because there is so much to say. I'm slowly regaining my inner strength that was there all along, but I had it tucked away due to my chronic state.

Whose hands are Lyme disease patients in? The doctors, the pharmaceuticals, the majority of doctors I've seen in the past twelve years have been ironic, to say the least. Most doctors are interested in only the dollar sign, the number of patients they can see, and the drugs they can prescribe. Of course, they get kickbacks from the pharmaceutical companies too.

Lyme disease is becoming a battleground in a national debate over treatment protocols; it's enough to make your head spin.

I feel as though Lyme disease is a conspiracy against us; as long as we stay ill and keep going from doctor to doctor, trying to determine what is wrong with us, they are making a fortune off us. They keep our bodies loaded with drugs, anything that they can prescribe for us, ordering up test after test as they try and figure it out.

I've had to learn a great deal and I've taken a few hard fall backs on finding a doctor who was willing to help me. I've learned how to recognize and respect Lyme disease for the seriousness that it is. I find I often take better care of others before myself in an unselfish way. It saddens me, though, that I have somewhat abandoned my siblings and friends. It's easier to just keep to myself and focus on the now. I would much rather talk to my friend, Lotus, the Pug she doesn't question me or judge me for what I can or cannot do in life; she loves me unconditionally.

Lyme disease is a devastating disease, but when you finally get the proper diagnosis, you can cope with it; it's the not knowing of what's wrong with your health. It twisted my mind, my body, and my emotions like a rope, entwined over and over again into a huge knot of disbelief and mistrust.

Lyme disease has its rewards. It has changed me; I have had to rely on myself, my self-doubts, my feelings on how and what I'm going to need to do to get through this. Because I know from all the research I have done in the beginning and all the physicians I had spoken to in the US and surrounding countries, plus the other Lyme disease victims, that I was in for hell of a battle.

This disease hasn't been a walk in the park for me, and I've suffered dearly with it, but with God's help I know I can do it now! God has graciously given me twelve years of life; he steadies me, he's listening, and he's given me the courage to speak up about Chronic Lyme disease and to try to get it acknowledged. Some days I hurt so badly and can barely walk upright, but I will not give in to this disease. My mind is so overloaded that I have a difficult time sleeping at night. I start to think about everything, all the stuff I want to say, be it positive or negative; my mind and my body are twisted with being objective and forthright of what I need to do and how I need to say what's on my mind.

It's amazing that I'm still alive so that I can tell you about this journey I'm on. Most of the doctors I know now and even my therapist can't believe I can even walk and exist. If you looked at my track record on my healthcare and my x-rays, you would understand. They have said repeatedly to me, "How do you even move? You have the body frame of an eighty-year-old woman!" Well, sometimes I wonder that myself! When I feel I'm at the end of my rope, I get another shot of energy. I guess I'm like a cat that has nine lives. I had better be careful—I may have already used them up. Oh dear!

I have been told by my Lyme disease doctor that it takes a long time to recover from having Lyme disease, but remember, I also have Rocky Mt. Spotted Fever. We don't even know how long I had that either. The good Lord only knows how long I've had it, the same with the Lyme disease. My Lyme disease doctor said, "It takes a long time to recover, if at all!"

We need to protect our Lyme-literate doctors who care for us and protect their rights as a physician to give us quality medical care. Isn't this what we should all be striving for—good medical care? Is anyone listening? How long will it take to bring attention to this matter? How many lives will be lost to this crippling death trap known as Lyme disease? When are we going to get this disease recognized and on the record? When can I open up a newspaper or a magazine and see the topic of Lyme disease and have discussions about it? The only time I see Lyme disease mentioned is on ways to prevent infection; well, I want more! I want to see articles on the chronic disease and how disturbing Lyme disease is and what victims have gone through to finally get a proper diagnosis. I want to see personal stories of the struggles that Lyme disease patients have gone through and the harassment that doctors have put these patients through. I want debates on Lyme disease. I want this out in the open once and for all!

The public healthcare systems and the news media need to learn the facts of preventative methods, better detection, better treatments, and help us Lyme disease victims find a cure.

The rights of patients and our treating physicians are being trampled upon by governmental and insurance agencies telling us it's "all in our heads". Luckily today, there are millions who are showing the world how wrong they are. This epidemic is being repeatedly spread throughout the U.S. and surrounding countries.

I'm also disgusted with comments from our mainstream medical and our caretakers who make comments like, "You look fine. Maybe you're just depressed." I've had comments made to me such as, "We all have to die of something, sometime." How callous are those words?

I can't let my guard down. I have to remain steadfast and keep a grip on my emotions. I need to keep some form of balance or normalcy for my husband as well. In one aspect, I'm thankful that I am the one with Lyme disease. I know I can handle this, my faith is holding me together. I feel God is testing me as to how strong a person I was, am, and will be. God will have his hands full, that's for sure!

Learn to get in touch with your inner silence and know that everything in this life has a purpose—a beginning and an end. I continually ask God to give me grace for today. Take a look at life, give thanks, accept your circumstances, give thanks, count your blessings that you're still alive, and give thanks!

You can set your sails, pull the anchor, cast away, feel the wind at your back, keep your eyes on the horizon, or stay on shore. It's your choice.

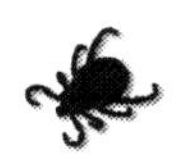

Treatment Options:

ALTERNATIVE VS. CONVENTIONAL

In 2001 I stopped using the antibiotics for Lyme disease and decided to try a different route. I used antibiotics for four and a half years and, yes, they helped me tremendously. But I had gone to thirteen doctors, three hospitals, and all the other medications plus antibiotics I have consumed in that period of time was nothing short of overwhelming. Then, when I was finally diagnosed, I was introduced to other antibiotics.

Many medical doctors are very leery of alternative therapies; some even say they're dangerous. But many of them are realizing that alternative treatments and the right approach are quite valuable. In today's medical realm, more and more alternative therapies are coming into focus. I feel that the mainstream medical community doesn't have all the answers and that is why I've studied and researched other avenues for my own benefit. I have learned and experienced many alternative protocols and, yes, you have to be careful and cautious of the alternative methods, as I found out.

But there are other alternative protocols that I am using today with the help of a wonderful doctor who is making a great impact on my health and my life. I have tried chiropractic, yoga, massage therapies, electro dermal, acupuncture, homeopathy, ayurveda, Chinese medicine, naturopathy, herbalists, aromatherapy, meditation, music therapy, nutritional therapies, qigong, and tai chi.

Some people choose one therapy and stick with it; others will start with one approach, and if that doesn't work, try another one. This is the approach I fell into with alternative therapies. I wasn't sure which therapy to try first. I was skeptical about doing alternative treatments but curious enough to try. I mean, after all, what did I have to lose? I knew my own family doctor would not be in favor of me doing this, and the other problem is it would not be covered by my insurance. Using alternative therapies is an out-of-pocket expense.

I made an appointment with a homeopathic doctor in a nearby town, scared out of my mind but very anxious to see what she could do or offer me in a way of balancing out my life. I couldn't handle the conventional treatments for the Lyme disease; I needed a change of treatments. That's when I was slowly introduced into another world of vitamins and supplements to replace the conventional medications. The price of these vitamins was costly, I would soon find out. The initial cost of starting this alternative therapy was $205, the practitioner had me do a patient history and electro dermal screening (a form of acupuncture) to evaluate the imbalances in my system. They uncovered a wide array of health conditions, including allergies, asthma, flu, arthritis, as well as my having Lyme disease and Rocky Mt. Spotted Fever.

She scheduled me for every month for six months, and then she introduced me to homeopathic remedies as follows:

FIRST MONTH:

(FATIGUE, DEPRESSION, ARTHRITIS, LIVER AND IMMUNE SYSTEM)

Pulsatilla 200c, 3 pellets once a day (nerves)

Enviro Detox 2 sprays , 3 times a day

SAME liquid 1 tsp. under the tongue

Acidophilus (yeast buildup)

Evening Primrose (Immune & Female Hormones)

Bromelain (Pain)

B150

Melatonin Sublingual (sleep)

**Used all of these for one month, didn't see much improvement.*

SECOND MONTH:

ENVIRO DETOX 2 SPRAYS, 2 TIMES A DAY

Myosis Nosode drops, 10 drops 3 times a day

SAME liquid 1 tsp. 2 times a day

Complex 2 tsp. 2 times a day

Now head relief up to 9 tsps. Per day

Mega B (all the B vitamins)

Melatonin

1–3 day juice fast ending with a Candida diet

I felt better but nothing great to report. Then three weeks later, I started a Candida diet to help heal the body. Sugar is a bad thing; it feeds the bacteria.

I pictured all this in my mind—here we go folks, think about this now: when you sprinkle a package of dry yeast over warm water, it starts to bubble and swell up. Well, imagine loading your system with sugar and the Lyme disease bacteria in your body spreads and grows like the yeast on the water. Not a very pretty thought and quite intimidating!

My diet consisted of vegetables, nuts, seeds, whole grains, fish/shellfish, poultry, dairy, red meats, butters, fats, beverages. Note: no fruit, no sugar!

> Example: Breakfast Sweet potato with walnuts, water
> Lunch Beets and spinach with fresh lemon, water
> Dinner Quinoa, steamed cauliflower and zucchini, water
> If you need a snack, eat more walnuts and carrots and
> Lots of water

I began to question myself. What did I get myself into? Of course, I was told if you get hungry, you can freely eat or graze on more vegetables throughout the day.

To say the least, this diet was a killer to be on. After weeks of doing this diet, I went back to her office so she could reevaluate how my system was doing—not so great! I continued to shift into low gear, and I felt like I was dying of starvation! Then it was time for a follow up, and more homeopathic medicines were introduced to me.

There was Libido Stimuli (sexual functions) 1 tsp. 2 time a day

Biochemical Phosphates (leg cramps) 4 tablets before bedtime

Hi Stress B & C

Psyllium Husks (liver cleanse)

For heaven's sake, with all the vegetables and grains I was consuming, why do I need to cleanse my body? After all, I was already pooping through the eye of a needle, how much more do you want? Needless to say, you can imagine how much money I went through.

I ended up in July 2001 back at my Lyme disease doctor for conventional medications. What was going to be my next route of defense, treatment protocols, I had no idea. I felt awful; I'd spent a fortune on an alternative route that I had high hopes would somehow come together and work in my benefit so I could see a great change in my overall health. I was sadly mistaken; this was just the beginning for me of my hit-and-miss scenarios. I would pay the ultimate price for having Lyme disease all because the mainstream medical community didn't do their job in the beginning.

I had researched on the Internet about an MD, PhD, Lewis Mehl-Madrona who was the author of a book called *Coyote Medicine: Lessons from Native American Healing*. Here was a trained physician who gave up a lucrative private practice to embrace the Native American healing arts from his ancestors to integrate both ancient and modern medicine. I had been researching and entered chat rooms on the Internet asking about Native American treatments for Lyme disease in hopes of finding an answer to my problems.

I had read about sweat lodges and how they can purify one's system. So I proceeded to learn as much as possible about Dr. Madrona's therapy protocols.

Here is a man, a physician, who against all odds took it upon himself to pass on a light to his readers and patients to give back the compassion that our mainstream medical community has lost touch with, what is real and what is sacred about being human.

I found a Web site for this wonderful physician, so I emailed him. Dr. Madrona emailed me and discussed his thoughts on healing and what I was dealing with. He told me that healing is a special journey—people *can* get well. But before a person can do so, he or she must undergo a transformation of lifestyle, emotions, and spirit. I knew this would be a problem for me. I couldn't very well change my lifestyle; I was on a rollercoaster with emotions; and at the time I wasn't attending a church. I understood what Dr.Madrona was trying to convey to me: the vital role of story in health and healing. Dr. Madrona spoke to me about my illness and told me that illness has a spirit or soul. He also discussed relaxation, visualization, and storytelling. He then asked me if I had other diseases besides the Lyme, and I told him I had Rocky Mt. Spotted Fever. He also was not surprised of the length of time it took to get a proper diagnosis.

Native American medicine has been practiced on this continent for at least ten thousand years. This continent was a healthy planet; plagues and epidemics soon changed when the Europeans arrived. Native American methods attained long-term survival and avoided chronic diseases.

The conventional therapies have ignored their intention to heal patients; we've lost the power of belief and faith that all things are possible with God's intervention. We are a controlled society and are falling by the wayside, slowly destroying our healthcare and our planet. Native American healers have developed a combined therapeutic approach. It takes time to start a healing journey. Their approach is to concentrate on the individual's needs and multiple hours of understanding your individual thought processes.

We've been taught to ignore our emotions; it has become secondary. We are hurried in this society since the faster we go, the more money we can make. In the days before modern pharmaceuticals, "rest" was a key ingredient of any type of therapy. Healing requires time, this is disturbing to many because it wreaks havoc with our routines and bad habits that we have developed.

When you have a chronic illness, there's purification necessary for your body. I was most intrigued with the sweat lodges, and I was interested in learning how this process worked. But I was concerned with where I would go, what it involved, how would I get there, how long would I need to stay there and, of course, would my insurance cover any of this and would I be able to afford to pay out of my pocket?

I have read and studied the effects of using a sweat lodge and how it purifies your body. The healing secrets of Native Americans intrigue me greatly. Like a native spa, sweating symbolizes rebirth, and cleanses your mind and body; sweating also removes toxins. When you pour water over hot rocks, it offsets stress, fatigue, muscle, and joint pain.[13]

Although I was not ready to pursue the treatment from Dr. Mehl-Madrona, I appreciated his honesty and his insight.

Two thousand and one was not a very good year. My father-in-law died that year and this proved to be a very stressful time. Just what I didn't need, more stress! I'd never felt so alone in my life. I missed my father-in-law; after my dad died in 1978, I looked to my father-in-law to replace the loss of my own father. I learned a great deal from this man and I miss him dearly! There isn't a day that goes by that his name is mentioned or a thought comes to my mind of our friendship and the time I had with him while he was alive. In August 1, 2000, I ended up back in Dr. N's office with the flu; a urinalysis was performed. I had already gone to Dr. W at the eye clinic for a routine check up, due to having difficulties with my vision, macular dry eye syndrome. I also returned to my Lyme disease doctor, who ordered up more blood work, CBC's, electrolyte panels, glucose, BUN, and creatinine. I went to the lab to have blood work and then returned to Dr. N so we could figure out our next approach. The antibiotic that I was using was not working. My medical doctor does not seem to understand the complications with having Lyme disease. He ended up sending me in for more lab work, lipid functions, LDL/HDL, and hepatic function panels.

I ended up back at the eye doctor for more vision complications, back to the lab for more blood being stripped from my veins. The next thing I know, Dr. N tells me I'm developing hypertension.

I ended up back at my doctor coughing up blood, having chest pains, and he orders up Guaifenesin 600mg, only to find out I didn't have hypertension. My poor husband was developing hypertension over this ordeal with me.

In 2002 I began taking Wellbutrin for my nerves because I was so depressed and moody all the time. I don't know how my husband could put up with me or stand being around me back then. I had uncontrollable outbursts of anger, frustration, and moodiness. I was bouncing back and forth with finding the correct antibiotic.

In April, I ended up at Warren Radiology for a chest PA/LAT. PA test film is shot from the patient's back (posterior) through the chest to the front (anterior) of the chest. LAT test is usually shot from the left side and also the right side[14]. I was short of breath, irritable, had clammy hands and Dr. N thought it was my heart. He was great at ordering up tests for one thing or another; he'd tell me, "It's just routine," and I'd say, "Whatever!"

In May, I was ordered tests again: Echocardiography, Doppler Echo, Color Flow, Velocity; this was enough to make my head spin. Okay, Dr. N, enough is enough and like usual all those tests, blood work, and x-rays came back the same, normal, nothing showed up, the results were always the same.

I proceeded to telephone my attorney to see how she was doing with my disability and if she was having any headway with winning the case for me. It took five years for my attorney to win a disability case for me. I knew I wasn't going to work anymore; I wanted my life to go back to how I was before all this happened, but I knew my life was definitely going to change, and not for the better.

While I was seeing Dr. N, he gave me injections, flu vaccinations, tried to alleviate the allergies and congestion in my lungs that I always seemed to be afflicted with. I was scheduled for another x-ray, and the doctor had discovered fluid in my lungs and fluid on my knees. The radiologist stated, "You need support hose." I was then placed on Bumex, a water pill. It decreases the amount of water retained in the body by increasing urination. It is used to treat fluid retention in the lungs or swelling of hands and feet (edema) or HBP. The side effects may cause headaches, nausea, muscle cramps, weakness in my left side in the left shoulder all the way into my left foot. Even to this day, I still have daily bouts with this problem.

The side affects of these drugs are horrendous, and I feel they do more damage to your body than the disease itself. I continued on and in May I was back at my Lyme disease doctor trying another antibiotic, Dynabac, used to treat various infections. The side effects may cause indigestion, nausea, gas, stomach pains, headaches, and dizziness may occur.

I began to combine Lorabid with the Dynabac; at least those two combinations seem to be working together so far. I continued using the Wellbutrin and Zyrtec to keep the mood swings and the allergies at bay. Of course, my Lyme disease doctor encouraged me to use Mega B150, Acidolophilus, Potassium, and Red Yeast Rice along with the medicines.

No menses yet, sleep deprivation is becoming a problem. I'd be totally exhausted, lie down in bed and just could not fall asleep. I tossed and turned, kept waking up my husband, had restless leg syndrome, would come downstairs and drink numerous cups of sleepy time tea, sit and read, then pray to God to go to sleep. Go back to bed, two hours later, it would start all over again.

I managed to wake up and prepare breakfast for my husband, go back to bed, and sleep for two to three more hours. I would wake up with muscle spasms in my arms, my hands would atrophy, stress levels are rising, and cramping in my legs. I had to go in again for blood work then felt a little better.

The following day I was nauseated, achy, having another rough day, on edge, and feeling hopeless. My husband would ask me to go out maybe just to Wal-Mart; I think he felt bad that I wasn't getting out in the world enough. We would stop and usually eat supper, and I felt a little better. When the evening came, sleep was a problem again; I kept my husband awake, too hot, too cold, ached all over, not interested in lovemaking.

I was tired. I had to force myself to do just about everything in the house. My bones ached, my desire for much of anything is dwindling. I started having dizzy spells, right foot wouldn't support me, stumbled around, I was walking with a stick. I was too embarrassed to be seen with a cane; why, I don't know the answer. I was becoming despondent, fatigued, nervous, frustrated, and depressed. My husband asked me to go sailing to get me out of the house, so I decided to go. It was exhausting, it took me a week and a half to recover from a four-hour sail, and I didn't even do anything to help sail the boat.

The next day I was dead on my feet, wiped out, cancelled Dr. J's appointment, had aching hands and feet, was trembling and couldn't sleep. I finally gave in and called my Lyme disease doctor back and told him my symptoms. He was upset with me, "Why didn't you come to my office? Why didn't you call me? I can't help you if you don't come in to see me!"

The drug Cefzil was causing stomach pain, diarrhea, loss of appetite, nausea and vomiting. I move like a turtle, and I was beginning to look like one—wide across my rump! My knees hurt; I had difficulty with walking, was restless, stiff, and very tired. This is how it goes, you can feel really bad for a long time and then you have some really good days. The goal is to have better days and not as many bad ones. Finally, a good night's sleep prevails upon me. I made an appointment to go to Casal's Spa & Salon for a hair treatment because I was starting to feel more like myself and I wanted to look better.

I never get my hopes up because it can backfire at any given moment. It's like four steps forward and six steps backward. One afternoon I was watching my granddaughter, Monet, and we were upstairs putting change in her Poppy's glass jar and some of the change fell on the floor. I said "Monet, pick those up for Gramma," and with her tiny, little voice she replied, "But Gramma, I can't," and I said "Why not?" and she replied, "I have bad knees!" I thought I would die laughing at her. She has seen me get down on the floor with her and play and then realized I can't get back up.

This disease is strange how it manifests itself; it goes from one area of the body to the next, you never know what's going to be affected. Then the disease goes into hiding and you'd never know anything was wrong. A few months go by and I'm feeling good, no pain, sleep is improving; oh, I believe I can handle this now!

Uh, oh, I spoke too soon ... As I said, there are setbacks. My right foot is so numb, I wasn't sure if I had a foot down there. I'm falling over more and more, the stress is pushing all the wrong buttons again, I'm trying not to fret over everything. I'm not too social anymore, either. I get very nervous when I have to talk around people, I try to avoid conversations, my memory is at a void, I can't remember much about my childhood or my children's childhood, just bits and pieces. My brain knows what to say, but my mouth can't quite express what I'm thinking.

Oh land sakes, my menses have started; this proves to be quite difficult. Women who have Lyme disease around this time can have some severe bouts with the disease. I've been in the emergency room twice around this time of the month when I started having menses. This ordeal made me violently ill at times.

My allergies are annoying: wheezing, sore, and itchy throat. Dr. N put me on an Advair inhaler but forgot to tell me that you need to gargle after you use it. Oh, my throat was so sore at times I could barely eat or swallow. I stopped using the inhaler and everything cleared on its own.

I started listening to Joyce Meyer Ministries, reading my Bible, praying, and feeling much better. My right foot is swollen, hurts to walk on, so I sit and prop it up. I have all this pain on the right side, even my right ear, eye, and right side of my head is killing me. The next day it moved over to my left side: left side of my head, eye, ear and all the way down to my left foot. Those nasty organisms are swimming around in my blood and saying, "Ok, guys, let's see what damage we can cause her today!"

I went back to Dr. N. He said, "Your allergies are acting up and your sinuses are backed up. I'll put you on Humibid Decongestant and a nasal spray." I felt some relief, but boy, did my back hurt from this.

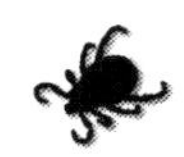

Battling for Disability

We finally have a ray of light from my SSD lawyer in December 2003! She sent me a letter saying she needed all my medical releases and to please sign below. I was excited over this; after all, I hadn't worked in three years and the doctors made it quite clear that I wasn't going to return to employment at all. They said I would not work outside my home again.

Dr. N lined me up to see a neurologist because of the difficulty with walking, paralysis in my right foot, and periodic numbness in legs and arms. The neurologist asked me, "When did you have shingles?"

I told her, "Last year, why?"

She stated, "I can see why on your left side of your hip across to the inner leg to your left knee you have no feeling, and when I applied pressure to your left leg, you nearly came off the table." Yes, that is true enough. She also stated, "I can't understand how you even move; you have some serious nerve damage on both sides."

My attorney called and told me they were waiting for a hearing with SSD benefits. "Please hang in there. I'm doing everything possible to get you some assistance. I pray that you are feeling better. I feel so badly for you that you are going through this, and I know that soon we'll get you some benefits." I told her the medicines and the doctor bills were so expensive and some of the drugs I couldn't afford to purchase because my insurance wouldn't cover them.

My attorney informed me, "If the judge, for some unforeseen reason, does not see you, I could file a Discrimination Suit against them," but I declined! My attorney was very persistent, she called and had reports from all the doctors I was seeing, she even went to the lengths of calling Congressman Ryan to have him check on Public Law 106–117 for me to see if I would qualify for it. The government is very political on who gets SSD and why. It isn't fair, but there's not much I can do about this now.

I started on new antibiotics; after taking them I was very nauseated. I had a very rough week and weekend, slept a great deal, was not interested in much of anything. I was resting and called my sisters and brother, which was the first step to actually carrying on a conversation. I felt a little better, did some cooking and baking, but was very tired yet.

I try to visit with positive people and talk occasionally with others on the phone, but this proves to be a difficult task for me. I stopped the antibiotics for a couple of days just to see if I would stop hurting. It did stop, but I went back on them and the pain started all over again. We decided to stop using the antibiotics on May 28, 2003. My family doctor wanted me to try Methaltrexate (Rheumatoid Arthritis drug) and Methycobalamin (derived from Vitamin B) injections everyday for three to six months. I declined to use those drugs. I wanted to wait and see what would happen from being off the other drugs.

I ended up back in Dr. J's office again with complications, he studies over the medical report from Dr. N and concludes his thoughts. "I believe Dr. N's diagnosis that you are sliding backwards again, the antibiotics you were using were causing liver pain and your liver enzymes are extremely high right now. I will stop the usage of them and see what transpires."

I am presently off the medicines, having difficulty with walking, headaches, joint pain and the fatigue continues. Dr. J informs me, "You are doing okay with no major complaints. Your exams for your heart and lungs are clear, abdomen is non tender, extremities with no edema, neuro is intact. I want you to stay on the medications I have you taking now and see if it makes a difference, and then I will follow up on how you do. Hopefully those changes we made will help you."

The problem with using antibiotics is we have no timelines to when to stop using them. My Lyme disease doctor isn't able to determine when and for how long to stop using them. Patients can vary with symptoms and have complications while using antibiotics; sometimes they become ineffective or you can develop rashes and then you need to stop the treatment. That's when you can determine yourself if you can handle being off them. There are signs and everyone reacts differently to this. So we take a break and see what develops. Some patients have been off antibiotics for five years or longer, are in remission, and doing just fine. Some of us aren't that fortunate, like myself. I stopped using the antibiotics, and I only can hold out for about two years when I need to go back to using the antibiotics. I develop complications with my respiratory system, and that's usually when I will go back to using them for a brief spell to knock down the Lyme in my system.

I ended up back at Dr. J's office again to try another antibiotic. He put me on Biaxin 50mg, 2 pills daily, Ativan 0.5mg, Diflucan 50mg and the Percocet 5/325mg. She gave me a list of the vitamins she was using from a holistic doctor, eleven different vitamins and supplements. I will not discourage her at this point; if she feels it's helping her then so be it.

In 2004 my attorney called and prepared me for my court arrival in front of the judge. "Please bring all your medical records, prescriptions, vitamins, and supplements along with you." My husband borrowed a handcart to take along with us so we could carry the above mentioned items. I had two boxes of medicine, three boxes of vitamins and supplements, a huge stack of medical records, receipts, and unpaid bills neatly tied all together on my handcart. My husband, me, and our neatly packed handcart arrived at the court office.

We sat in the waiting room with our number in hand, waiting for my review. My attorney came in and asked me for my handcart and off she went rolling it down this long hallway and then disappeared. We sat there for another two hours and then I heard my attorney come up to me and say, "Janet, this is it. Please come with me!"

I said, "Can David come along too?" She politely said, "No, they just want to see you, my dear!" My husband had to help me stand up on my feet because I was so stiff and sore I could barely move.

My attorney glanced at my husband smiled, winked, and told him, "Everything looks good." I didn't realize it at the time what that meant.I hobbled down this long hallway with my attorney at my side, and into the courtroom we went. There was this judge sitting up there in a huge platform, my attorney, there were two other doctors, one was a medical doctor and the other one was a psychologist that I never met before, and the court recorder was there and I felt I was going to pass out.

I was terrified; the judge had his secretary give me a glass of water to help calm me down. My attorney held my trembling hand; those two doctors started their representation for me. I'd never known doctors like this who cared, stood up, and fought for my disability like those two did.

They informed the judge, "Janet has Chronic Lyme disease. She is not going to improve, she will never be able to hold a job, her medical expenses have been astronomical and will continue to be, her life has been a living hell, and her life will be a chain of events and illnesses that will continue on until the disease itself takes her life. As you can see by her personal handcart that she brought with her, she has lost nine years of her life to a disease that should have been diagnosed properly. The outcry of unjustified medical treatments has weighed heavily on her, her husband, and her children. This is a disgrace to our country what this woman and countless of other men, women, and children are dealing with. Yes, Your Honor, she needs help financially to take the burden off her shoulders and her husband."

I just sat there in a "Lyme fog," this is not really a medical diagnosis, it's mainly derived from our toxic environment, heavy metals, insecticides, pesticides they are everywhere. Stress has a great deal of influence when it comes to lyme fog and how we feed our bodies is another aspect of lyme fog. It causes unclear thinking, trouble concentrating, forgetfulness and even felt(el) detached from (my) your body. I had to make changes by giving more responsibility to my husband, David when it came to helping him with his business. I wasn't able to concentrate and focus on doing the bookkeeping. I posted notes all over my refrigerator to remind me to take care of the banking and how to do the banking, making sure the bills were sent in the mail, what I was having for dinner I couldn't even understand the recipe and how to follow it. I learned how to avoid certain foods such as white sugar, white flour, sodas and sweets. I learned that certain exercises could help with the brain fog such as yoga, meditation and relaxation therapies, aerobics, walking and balance. I also learned to use vitamins such as B vitamins, Coenzyme Q10 and L-carnitine. The doctors shook my hand, and I was in shock! I don't believe I even knew at that time what really happened in that room on that day. As the judge's gavel came down on his desk, I felt like I was on a sinking vessel. He smiled at me, the doctors smiled at me, my attorney had a smile on her face. My attorney, my personal handcart, and I came walking back through the long hallway and up the corridor. My husband was waiting for me. My attorney said, "It's all over for her. She passed with flying colors!" My husband was so happy and relieved! I believe I was in shock that this entire morning I had the most remarkable, amazing doctors who stood with me and not against me, and fought a long, arduous battle for all Chronic Lyme disease patients all over this country. I was awarded disability and placed on Medicare A & B. As I said, those two doctors, one a medical and the other a psychologist stood in front of the judge and fought not just for me but for all Lyme disease victims. My insurance company was relieved that I wasn't with them anymore.

My insurance company was enthralled that I finally was off their ledger.

I had signed up for water therapy at the YWCA two weeks later after recovering from my cold.

I returned to Dr. N because I wasn't getting any better. He told me, to "Stop using the Ryna-twelve." He gave me samples of Claritin 1 per day, took my blood pressure and it was 118/70. My sinuses were drying up although I still had coughing spells to the point where I'd vomit.

Dr. N asked me about the Lyme disease, I told him I was having muscle spasms, ache(d) all over and tired, numbness in my hands and arms, memory lapses, moody, back pain, leg pain, stabbing sensations in my ears and eyes, speech problems, and a creeping weight gain.

My husband suggested maybe I could get a personal trainer for a couple of days a week along with my water therapy. I had a young man who helped me with low impact stretching and strengthening my muscles. I continued on with the water therapy and my personal trainer. I was researching and reading all information available and that I could get my hands on. I was in dire straits to find another way of treating this Lyme disease instead of the antibiotics. My body just couldn't handle them anymore.

My older brother, Tommy, died on March 22, 2004 from cancer, although I'm not exactly sure what kind. He had tumors in various places in his body, his adrenal system, lung, and a brain tumor. I was very depressed and angry. I knew Tommy would be in heaven with Marg and Doyle; they would all be free of pain and at peace.

My husband and I decided I'd had enough of the antibiotic and it was time to make a change. Before my brother died, he was seeing a naturopathic doctor for his back pain and seemed to be quite taken with him. So I decided that I'd make an appointment with him and see what he could do for me. At that particular time in my life, I had a great deal of difficulty with dressing myself. So I would lay my pants on the floor, sit on the edge of the bed, and inch my feet into my pants. Then my husband would help pull my pants up for me. My husband then would assist me in walking down the stairs and help me into our car.

My husband and I went into his office for an appointment, and we were amazed at how many people were there seeking his help and getting it. It's unlike any doctor's office I've ever been to—very laid back. I felt like I was at a family reunion instead of a physician's office. Everyone was talking about their health situations and laughing; it was rather comforting instead of a cold, unfeeling office where you're observed and ignored by the staff and by other patients. Not so here!

This doctor had a whole new approach to health care. We talked and told him about my situation and all my health problems. Dr. S focused on helping me to restore balance to my body, helping me to resolve my health problems, and he showed me how to reach my goals in attaining better health. He doesn't believe in drugs and surgeries; he believes in finding the problem and fixing it, not masking or just treating the symptoms. He recognizes that each individual has an imbalance someplace in their body, and he tries to discover what it is and then does his best to fix it.

Dr. S has over twelve years of experience in a field known as "Holistic Healthcare." I wish I would have known he was around nine years ago; maybe I wouldn't be in the predicament I'm in now today. Lessons I learned from this doctor has given me a new outlook on my own healthcare. I cannot believe his approach to healthcare and what a difference it has made for me and my life. I actually felt as though my life was over while seeing the mainstream medical community and meeting this educated, honest physician.

Dr. S is a licensed naturopathic physician (ND) and is educated in all of the same basic sciences as a medical doctor but also studies holistic and non-toxic approaches to therapy with a strong emphasis on disease prevention and optimizing wellness. Dr. S is expertly trained in clinical nutrition, acupuncture, homeopathic medicine, botanical medicine, chiropractic, and he encourages patients to make lifestyle changes in support of their personal health.

Naturopathic medicine concentrates on whole-patient wellness and the medicine is tailored to the patient and emphasizes prevention and self-care. Naturopathic medicine attempts to find the underlying cause of the patient's condition rather than focusing solely on symptomatic treatment. Dr. S cooperates with all other branches of medical science referring patients to other medical doctors for diagnosis or treatment, when appropriate.[15]

Now I have some wonderful doctors I still see who are not Naturopathic doctors, but they are willing to work alongside my ND, and we manage quite well together in my best healthcare.

Dr. S's approach to preventative healthcare isn't considered a one-time treatment. He outlines a wellness program for you and your health problems. There are steps that have to be taken over time to repair your health. The way you are today and the way you will be in the future is a vast result of what is in your past. All of us have inherited weaknesses, genetically speaking. We have all been exposed to daily physical, chemical, and emotional stresses. To develop and to maintain our health is a daily and life long effort.

And not everyone is cut out for this, like I said, you really, truly want to do this for your own peace of mind.

What a breakthrough it has been for me and can be for you too! From the time we are born, we should have been given the tools to prevent health problems and not wait until we suffer with symptoms and then our real problems begin. Our healthcare is "maxed out"—overwhelming expenses for prescriptions, insurance premiums, insurance for Lyme disease is unbearable for many.

Dr. S placed me on a program to detox my already toxic filled body as follows:

> Colon Care—a powdered mix that I added to apple juice followed by a glass of water. This was to eliminate the toxins in my system. Epican Forte—used to rebuild cells and tissues in my immune system and to promote normal cell growth. I took two tablets two times daily with food.
>
> Cat's Claw—to build up my immune system and help with arthritic pains. I took three tablets daily with meals.
>
> Ultra Stress—made with B complex, Vitamin C and Iron, once daily
>
> Coral Calcium—helps to build up whole body system for energy, four daily

I continued with this protocol, and I could not believe how satisfied I was and how wonderful I felt. And I was able to lose ten pounds, which made it all worthwhile!

When I visit my other doctors, they always comment, "So, Janet, what do you want me to do today?" When you have Chronic Lyme disease, you know so much more about the disease than the majority of doctors out there so you are kind of more in control of your own healthcare. My doctor's work well with me, and they have seen with their own eyes what and how I have improved since seeing Dr. S Maybe not in my time now, but maybe in the future, there could be a whole new approach for better medical care.

Dr. S planned out his healthcare assessment for me. He spoke of "structural balance," which means correcting your physical imbalances; "nutritional support," customizing a specific diet and nutritional supplements for your specific needs; "energy balance" to correct these energy and meridian or acupuncture blockages in your body.

The possibility of surgery with Chronic Lyme disease is at a very high rate due to other diseases that come on board with this disease. Luckily, with the help from Dr. S, I have been able to avoid these problems. He's helping me to reduce my pain and suffering, and I'm slowly learning to utilize a non-medical, natural approach to help restore my health. He is helping me to restore balance in my body, physical and nutritional aspects for my body. He is trying to restore my body back to "good health" without the use of drugs.

He recognizes my battle with Chronic Lyme disease and is doing everything in his heart and soul to give me a unique balance and to recognize me as an individual with compromising conditions, what my problems are and teaching me how to cope with this disease. What more can I ask for? It's the first time in twelve years I finally feel I can handle it, and I know with Dr. S's understanding and with God's help, I will prevail!

I went for X-rays on my spine and found I have spinal stenosis, bone spurs, herniated discs, and degenerative disc disease to compound my health problems along with the Lyme disease.

One of the primary modes of treatment is a technique called Flexion Distraction. He also used a technique called the distraction pump. We discussed nutritional values because the discs are degenerating.

Flexion Distraction is a technique which has become the most widely used approach to treating symptomatic disc injuries involving back pain and often accompanying leg pain. Flexion Distraction involves the use of a specialized table that gently distracts or stretches the spine and allows the chiropractor to isolate the area of disc involvement while slightly flexing the spine in a pumping rhythm. When I lay on this special table, the lower half of my body is gently moving up and down. There is no pain involved while I'm doing this.

The distraction pump is a hand-held instrument to help reduce disc herniation and relieve facet syndrome and spinal stenosis. This excludes pressure exerted on the peripheral nerves and associated tissues. I can feel the doctor's hand applying pressure on the areas affected on my back. There is minimal stretching and pressure, if any, placed on the nerves.

One of the key ingredients in his treatments for most people is patience! This condition did not develop overnight, and it will not go away overnight either. Following the treatments he planned out would need to be done precisely. Dr. S has helped me to get back up on my feet, walking and dressing myself. But it took a good three years to get to this point!

Learning to trust your instincts or your gut feelings, you'd be amazed at how your body speaks to you. It's important to pay close attention to your health; it helps with decision making, reducing stress, and improving your lifestyle.

Keeping a journal throughout this time has helped. It's given me a chance to improve and clarify my well-being and to define my overall health care. Learning to blend medicines and medicinal practices has been the best of all worlds. I have undergone many therapeutic and non-therapeutic practices throughout my twelve years, and I have experienced good and bad in all of the practices. I have nothing to lose; I was once healthy and now I am faced with a lifetime of chronic pain and disability. It was very depressing, to say the least, but now I know I can cope with it all. I feel that more and more mainstream medical practitioners will blend into the alternative state of therapies. I have read many articles and medical journals recording studies that alternative therapies have real value. But the real drive behind the natural and alternative methods are the people, consumers like myself and others. No one is forcing us to use them; it's just a good word-of-mouth support. I tell my family and friends of my pains and suffering and how much better I feel, how much better I look, and they can see for themselves the difference in me.

I never realized how much nutrition played a part in my recovery. Dr. S put me on a nutritional balance program. I thought I would die when he put me on this diet or change of eating. Dr. S only wanted me to eat veggies, fruits, no red meats, lean cuts of meat like chicken, turkey, fish, nuts and seeds, and lots of water. Dr. S told me to only eat what God has provided—sound advice and true!

As I continued on with Dr. S and his back treatments, we then decided to take a closer look at other areas of my healthcare. He had me fill out a health assessment of what I wanted to see, how important to find other areas of my healthcare to be acknowledged, what other problems I had and how to best fulfill those areas. After I did this, he laid out a program for me for nutritional supplements to help rebuild my immune system, bone strengthening, and to help me cope with it all emotionally, physically, and spiritually.

Through my experiences, I continued to write poetry.I wrote a poem about an oak tree in my front yard one afternoon because of my dependency on God for so much. I depended on Him (God) more than my own husband, children, other family members, and even my doctors. God has taught me and shown me that in his time, he will heal me.

THE RUGGED OAK TREE

As I sit here on my front porch
I wonder what will become of me.
So many thoughts are wondering
Thru my mind and thinking of eternity.
Oh I wonder and wonder what
Will my life come to be?
Will God look down and say
Dear Girl, do you ever think of me?
I look out over the front yard
At this stately old oak tree
The many ways that tree takes form
It takes its hold on me!
It showers me with strength and love
It's a pleasure to sit and look upon
But then I think of what the tree meant,
When it's cut down, what life and purpose does it represent?
When Jesus hung on an old wooden cross
Was it perhaps an old rugged oak tree?

I have to stay the course, trust in him, and just live one day at a time!

October 30th through November 5th, 2004, my medical doctor, Dr. N, sent me for a complete work up, metabolic panels (a comprehensive blood test that measures sugar levels, electrolytes, fluid balance and kidney functions) blood counts, coronary reactive protein, (CRP is a blood test that measures the amount of a protein called C-reactive protein in my blood). It measures general levels of inflammation. I suppose because I wasn't seeing my Lyme disease doctor, he wanted to make sure everything was going in the right direction.

I kept developing sinus and throat conditions, laryngitis, upper respiratory infections, and Dr. N would send me in for tests to determine what was going on and what his next step would be to treat me. I told Dr. N that while I was seeing Dr. S, his protocol was alleviating the pain, sleep problems, I had a little more energy, and his back treatments seemed to be effective.

Then it was off to the eye doctor to determine if the Lyme disease was damaging my eye tissue. I had bouts of dry eye irritations constantly, so he had me use artificial tears to keep my eyes lubricated. This curtailed my reading and researching on the Internet, books, and magazines was not good for my eyes. Even when I was outside, I could feel the strain. If the wind would be blowing around especially where I live, the prairie grasses, ragweed, goldenrod, dust, pollen all those wonderful factors would force me back into the house. There were many days that I couldn't open the windows or have the doors open, it was just too much of a strain.

I continued with my ongoing medical problems, solving one or two with only to resolve them and then later to experience other complications with having Chronic Lyme disease. I was still seeing Dr. S and doing my naturopathics and my back therapy to regain my strength and my balance. It was a long rough road coming back unsure of whether or not all of this therapy was going to pay off or not. I would question myself many times; my family was skeptical too. Fear was probably their driving force because of this unknown territory I was walking into. Why was it so difficult for them to understand that I needed reassurance and encouragement instead of being doubting Thomases? I have to give this doctor a chance to prove to me that it was all worthwhile.

I felt as though I was finally awakening my spirit to help me grow and to maybe find healing. I often would listen to Native American music, their chants, songs, and music traditions to give me peace and understanding. My love for music and voice has helped me cope with having Chronic Lyme disease. I enjoy all facets of music, and I enjoy singing. I suppose there have been many times people have seen me singing away in my truck. Sometimes people would smile, give me a thumbs up, toot their horn at me, and I'm sure others thought I was nuts. Who cares? I don't. I am so immersed in the music; it lifts me up no matter how bad I feel or how much pain I'm in. The music in my life has helped shape me into the person I am becoming. I'm trying to make a positive difference.

Dr. S has always encouraged me to reach a little further. I give this doctor credit for teaching me to speak up and learn about my health concerns and to take charge of my health and decision making when it comes to my own healthcare, not to leave it in the hands of the medical, but for me to be aware of what's going on and trusting myself to ask questions and finding the answers.

Having faith has really helped me too cope with this disease. We are all on a journey, and if by some unfortunate chance you are detoured because of an illness, it makes the journey even more challenging to stretch out your arms and embrace the beauty that surrounds us. Whether you embrace music or artistic endeavors, just embrace life, give homage to your relationship with your God in your own way and in your own surroundings.

I've read numerous books on the health benefits of laughter and how it can relieve stress. Laughter can stimulate your immune system and increase the capacity to fight disease. When I laugh, I think about all those little spirochetes (Lyme bacteria) in my body running as fast as possible to get away from the laughter. These nasty little creatures do not want me to be happy; they want to keep me sick and miserable.

The majority of the medication in today's world can't do what laughter does, and with laughter you won't have to worry about side effects. One day, in December of 2008, I was speaking to my brother and we started talking about a game he played a long time ago with some friends. After he told me, I burst out in such a load roar of laughter, and then he was laughing so hard he had to excuse himself!

There is nothing more enjoyable than to hear babies or small children laughing; it evokes your own laughter and is quite contagious. I've laughed so hard with my granddaughter, Monet, that I had tears rolling down my face and my stomach would ache. My girls, when they were still living at home, would just start laughing for no reason whatsoever, and before long I felt like my gut would split open from laughing so hard. Yes, it is a good thing and makes you feel wonderful!

I ended up back in Dr. J.'s office to review my symptoms and to start another round of antibiotics for a while. Dr. J stated, "I had high hopes that you wouldn't need to see me again; you seemed as though maybe you were on the road to a remission. But being that I don't have a test to determine if you are in remission, it's difficult to say." He asked me about the fatigue, wanted to know my activities of the day and what they consisted of. I told him just my usual morning routine, waking up, starting breakfast for my husband, put a load of clothes in the washer and by that time my legs felt like Jell-O, so I'd lay down and sleep for a while. I woke up finish my laundry, take the dog for a walk, work around the house a little, then became short of breath, my heart would beat so hard I thought it would jump out of my pajamas. So I'd sit down and rest, read my Bible, read my scriptures, go down and work on the computer, fall asleep in my chair. I'd wake up again, start dinner early because I knew I'd be exhausted by the afternoon. I had pain that would generate in my neck and work its way down into my spinal area. I knew this would curtail any other activities.

Dr. J. wanted me to go to my family doctor and have tests performed on me to try and determine what was happening, again. I refused to go. I told him no way! I told Dr. J. that every test I go and have the results are the same, they're negative. We all know why nothing shows up on the test results—because it's the Lyme. On occasions I have found it necessary to have my health checked out, but nine times out of ten it's the same diagnosis—nothing—and then I know the Lyme disease is in control again. So I just live with it and keep going.

Dr. J. explained to me that my symptoms may be aggravated by activity, stress or weather conditions. I would tell him I was using natural medicines to help with the problems I was experiencing. He never disagreed about me using or seeing a ND, he rather encouraged it. He would give me other options to try, and I had to decide what I needed to do in order to alleviate the problems I was dealing with again. I used the antibiotic for a short period of time. I realized that the antibiotics at that particular time, I needed to give my body a break again. I spoke to my ND about my visit with my Lyme disease doctor, but you have to remember he doesn't believe in synthetic medications, only natural ones. He's a firm believer that medicines only cause more harm to your system.

So I continued to falter, and my dear husband thought I should be returning to Dr. J, my Lyme disease doctor, but I decided against his better wishes.

My daughter kept insisting that I should go and see a holistic doctor, Dr. M. So in 2005 I scheduled an appointment with Dr. M. I asked my mother-in-law to ride down with me to his office. It looked like at one time or another it may have served as a railroad station. I sat there in my car wondering if this was the place; it just didn't seem like a typical doctor's office. The address my daughter gave me was correct, and I was in the location she discussed with me prior, so we ventured into the office. I was rather surprised at what we saw inside the building: shelves with natural foods, refrigerators and freezers full of food; I thought I was standing in a health food store. Vitamins and supplements were stacked in every corner, but where was the doctor's office located? We sat down in the store, and in walked a very tall man; he didn't act like or look like a doctor that I was used to seeing. To say the least, I was terrified. I wanted to just get up and walk out, but I drove all this way down here, and my daughter just felt with certainty that he could help me. So being the mother that I am, I didn't want to disappoint her. I took a deep breath and sat down in his office. There were diplomas on his wall, and he had a portrait of Jesus, so I thought he must believe and have faith, so that was encouraging to me. Then I noticed all these machines on his desk, and beside his desk, black bands were lying beside this one machine that I soon would be using. It kind of reminded me of a movie about Dr. Jekyll, experimental in the dungeon, some type of torture machine.

We discussed my Lyme disease, Rocky Mt. Spotted Fever, everything I was going through, all the misdiagnosis, the doctors, tests, traditional medicines, natural medicines; we talked about my family, where I grew up and where I live now.

Then he asked me to place these long black bands (looked like big, wide rubber bands) over my wrists, and he then proceeded to hook them to a machine called a Cybernetic Biofeedback Xrroid Report of Naturopathic stressors, not meant to be construed as an Allopathic diagnosis of disease or illness. I felt like I was getting a lobotomy. I had no idea what he said to me, but I sat there with those bands around my wrists, and then I noticed all these tapes were printing off this machine and reports were printing on his printer beside his desk. My name was on the top of the report—the date, a two-column report with numbers 0–100, anything below 50 was considered okay, anything over 100 wasn't a good sign—malabsorption, body's not absorbing.

He then told me that the Lyme disease has set up an Immune Response. He explained I have pyrus pouches in my intestinal tract.

I thought this sounded kind of wacky. I was fearful that it might kill me in the end; I'd never heard of anything like this, but I put my trust in him.

On this report, it was broken down in all the different locations as minerals, amino acid, nutritional, B Vitamins, Tissue slats, Fatty acids, Vita K, Vita C, Vita D, Vita A, Overall Enzymes, Special reports on nutrition. I did find the reports extremely interesting, but I wasn't fully aware of the context and how he was able to get these numbers and how my body responded to them. But I did find it intriguing; I'd never experienced anything quite like this before.

The reports broke everything down and that was fascinating to me as well. Then he started to explain what my body was telling him.

SAMPLE REPORT:

1. Syndrome X-Vanadium (Liver & Kidney functions), Insulin Resistance—it's not acting and working the way it should; with this fatigue you have, your body is not able to bounce back like it should.
2. Degeneration in Nerves
3. K-3 Auto Immune Problem—overall enzymes, kidneys, and liver aren't able to compensate.
4. ACTH—Hormone & Kidneys
5. Malabsorption—body's not absorbing (6) Minerals, (5) Amino Acids, (2) Fatty Acids, and (6) Enzymes
6. Lactose Intolerant—Proteins, sugar, yeast
7. Insulin resistant
8. Body is not getting energy from anything, Mega Colon
9. Lacking certain vitamins, minerals, hormonal, protein, digestion—he told me I need to do this through foods, eat only slightly cooked vegetables three times a day.

Dr. M then proceeded to tell me that the Lyme disease was leaning toward cancer.

When I returned to Dr. S for a back treatment, I discussed Dr. M with him and his findings and I told him what Dr. M said about the Lyme leaning toward cancer. He was livid.

I went back to Dr. M and he told me not to give up, pray to God for strength, because it's going to take a great deal of strength and determination to overcome this. He also told me, "You've come this far. I'll do everything in my power to help you live a normal life. You will have setbacks, but you already know this! You need to stay on the diet Dr. S put you on and keep doing the treatments for your herniated discs. They are working for you and continue with Dr. S supplement and vitamins program."

Then Dr. M proceeded to tell me about Lyme disease and where it originated from and then proceeded to tell me that it's a biological warfare mistake. He also explained that Borellia is the sister and that Lyme disease is the brother, and he was going to weaken the sister to kill the brother.

I said, "Doctor, explain Lyme disease and biological warfare to me again." He said, "The U.S. had a truck loaded with biological warfare to make Lyme disease small enough, the government was going to release it in the Everglades, but the truck crashed in Lyme, Connecticut, and this is where it all started." I just sat there in a daze and couldn't believe what he told me ... Is this why Lyme disease is so misunderstood?

He then put me on a most probable natural approach, listed as follows:

Pituitary Pineal Hypothalamus drops 2x 10–15 drops daily
Quentakehl 5x 5–15 drops daily
Sanukehl Serra 6x 5–10 oral with bacterial involvement
Notrakehl 5x 5–15 oral drops
Utilin's 6x twice a day, 5 times a week (rub on)
Episcorit 2 drops 5 daily, oral
Cervikehl 2 drops 5–10 daily, oral
Toa Free Cat's Claw 2 drops 5–10 daily

These were small vials of liquids, and it was his way of treating the Lyme disease. Dr. M stated to me, "We will see what results your body shows after a while and how you respond to everything; then I'd like to put you on a natural drug to try and kill the Lyme."

As I stepped out of his office to pay for all of this ($282), I was asking myself, what in the world am I doing? God, give me strength because I pray all of this works for me. I went out to my car and just sat there stunned by everything that happened and what he said to me in his office. I just sat there in the car, and I was just in shock, I guess! I didn't know if what I was about to do here was worth $282, but I was pretty committed at that point in time. We drove home, and we stopped for a bite to eat so I could reflect on what had just happened. The next question out of her mouth was, "What do you think David is going to say about this?"

"I have no clue. I do know that he has never discouraged me or hindered me from trying new therapies, and he has always stood beside me on all of it." He may not always agree with me when I go on these tangent adventures, but he's seen me at my worst with fighting this disease. We are always open to new ideas and new thoughts about how to treat Lyme disease; it's a very complicated disease to have.

I do know that the majority of the "mainstream medical community" would not like how this doctor tested me to determine my health assessment. In fact, I had discussed this with my medical doctor, and he wasn't too supportive at all. I told him, "I do not want to go back to the traditional treatment for the Lyme disease and that is the antibiotic. I believe my body just cannot tolerate them anymore. I do believe, though, that the antibiotics helped me in the beginning, and I'm grateful to my Lyme disease doctor for what he did to help me along. I just want to try another avenue of natural treatments and see where this takes me. We arrived home with my bag full of tinctures, pills, and my interpretation cybernetic feedback, and my husband and I sat down to discuss this report from Dr. M. I told him everything he discussed with me and showed him all the bottles of pills and liquids that I was to use. I think I was more nervous about telling him *how* much it cost than anything else!

My husband was a little bit shocked, but I feel he just wanted to see some improvement with my healthcare and hopefully to get my life back. It's not been an easy ordeal for him, and he's seen me at my lowest point, where I wasn't sure if I was going to live much longer.

I started using my vials and taking it as scheduled on a daily basis. It was a few days before I noticed any differences in the way I felt. I found this to be another new challenge, but I also had to remember that it was not the end of the world. I had options on how I had to look at what I was doing, why I was doing this, and how I was going to handle it. I was using eight different holistic herbal vials and thirty drops from these tinctures up to three times a day. I myself was skeptical about this and what I put myself in and what may be the outcome from doing this. I hadn't noticed anything significant in the way I felt.

My pen and paper were on fire! I wrote down anything and everything. I have notes on the backs of paper bags, toilet paper, paper towels, wherever I was at the time. My journals, all of them, have been my constant companions, I was busy penning. We all have talents in one form or another, and how we choose to use them or express them depends on you. Either it be through designing, art work, music, or writing, it's knowing when and where to use these gifts. My writings have been a godsend for me; my imagination comes alive. In all actuality, it's much easier for me to write than to talk due to the uncertainty of speech, my speech patterns, and thought processes. I have a tendency to stutter over my words, and I can't think clearly sometimes. But most important creative energies have helped me to stay focused, a little healthier, and much happier.

We all need to look around at the truly amazing world we live in, nourish it, we can all appreciate the beauty around us, if we would just open our eyes, our hearts and our minds. We need to just look around at all of the amazement and try to live one day at a time, we're too hurried. Just put first things first, I'm trying to honor and respect myself through this journey that I'm on and I'm trying to stay close to God throughout this journey.

I took so much for granted before and I believe that God gives us these challenges when we are afflicted with an illness, it's what we do about it and how we choose to live with it that helps us to understand His purpose for our life, and being grateful despite the Lyme disease.

I continued to see Dr. M and used the natural medications he placed me on. I also continued to see Dr. S for my back treatments. Dr. S was doing allergy eliminations and my back and leg treatments twice a week.

On Dr. S treatment protocol, I was using Stress B, Organic Minerals, Flax Oil, Megaglymax, Liquid Iodine, Liquid Ashwaganda, and Liquid Rheumania; those three liquids I would mix in water one tsp. each day for one week. Those liquids were vile tasting, but they sure made a huge difference in my energy levels. It worked like a charm!

I was also using the conventional medications: Ativan (nerves), Clarinex (allergies), and Percocet (pain).

I started to develop a reaction to Dr. M.'s drops and came down with flu-like symptoms. I called him, and he informed me that this is a natural response until your body adjusts to the drops.

Dr. S was leery about Dr. M that I was also seeing and the vials he was using. He kept an eye on what was happening to me along the way.

I went back to Dr. M, and he proceeded to do another Cybernetic Test on me. I didn't like what I was seeing; it's unbelievable how much information comes from using these bands.

In May I went in again to see Dr. M, and he put the bands on my wrists again for my biofeedback report. "Janet," he said, "you have another variation (biological warfare) Bruccellosis. It's an infection caused by a bacteria passed among animals, namely sheep, goats, cattle, deer, elk, pigs, and dogs." Our daughters had raised a sheep and a goat, numerous deer roamed our property, and we had dogs.

Symptoms of this are fever, sweats, headaches, back pains, joint pains, and fatigue.

Ways to get it include eating, drinking, or breathing infected meat or contact with infected animal carriers.

Biological Warfare can be a potential use; also can be used by an aerosol route resulting in infection to mimic a natural disease.

Then he informed me that I had hypodrenia—weak adrenals,

which in turn he explained to me, adrenal insufficiency is usually caused by an autoimmune disease or by adrenal damage stemming from long-term use of cortisone. While I was seeing Dr. P for my back problems, he was injecting me with cortisone injections every week for one month at a time. This is why my bones were fracturing and why I had all of this scar tissue on my lungs from the overuse of cortisone. I was also getting cortisone injections for allergies and lung problems.

This was just the tip of the iceberg!

Dr. M's testing was revealing a series of health problems, hormonal imbalances, food allergies, environmental toxins, the role of sugar, was about to unfold in catastrophic anomalies.

Dr. M put me on Pineal Pituitary Drops one dropper per day and Cat's Claw one dropper two times a day. Only $98 later, I continued to use the drugs and had much more energy and was able to hold up a little longer throughout the day.

I continued with Dr. S for my back and allergy treatments, and he was keeping a close eye on my treatments with Dr. M. This went on for a few more months, and I seemed to be handling everything well, or so we thought. I scheduled myself to return to Dr. M for another biofeedback report, and the numbers seemed to be adjusting.

Dr. M performed another test on my Lyme disease, and his report came up with the Spotty Fatigue (RMSF), and once again he mentioned, Biological Warfare variations. So I said, "What else is new? My body is overloaded with biological warfare components, and I'm also loaded with inflammation in my body due to these infections with Chronic Lyme disease, RMSF, Brucellosis, so now what?"

Dr. M decided to try another step with my health care assessment. He placed me on MESO drops to continue with detoxing and helping with cellular repair and repairing my body. Then I started feeling strange with this new treatment. I was then beginning to question myself or perhaps stop this treatment protocol with Dr. M. I thought maybe it was time to have a heart-to-heart talk with God about all of this because I was scared to death and so overwhelmed over what was starting to happen to me.

I couldn't get it out of my mind—Dr. M telling me my body was full of biological warfare variations was terrifying. I noticed my personality was really being affected, and I didn't want to be around family members or even my friends. I was having a difficult time with dealing with my emotions. I felt like I was riding a rollercoaster but unable to get off of it; it just kept winding around in circles, up and down.

I found a prayer in the *The Power of Prayerful Living*[16] by Doug Hill and *God Take This Pain* by Marianne Williamson.

GOD, TAKE THIS PAIN

Dear God,
The pain of this life is more than I can bear.
I feel as though death would be better
My thoughts are dark, my sorrows huge
I feel as though I shall not endure, and
There is no one and nothing to turn to now.
My hurt is so big
I cannot handle this
If you can, dear God, please do
If you can, Please Do Amen.

I wrote that down and read that at every given moment I had. I felt my days were coming to a close end. I don't know if it was from all the natural medicines I was consuming or all these horrible toxins. I couldn't reach out to my family or friends. These are the ones who are supposed to love you and support you, the ones who will hang in there for the long haul. There were many in my family and friends who did not like this doctor, and they could tell he was harming me instead of helping me.

I went back to Dr. M, who put me on a natural drug (some type of cancer drug; I don't remember what it was) to try and snuff these diseases out. I was detoxing at the time, but with Dr. M's detox program I couldn't leave the house; my bowels just let loose.

I was watching Joyce Meyers, and she was talking about depression one morning. Joyce says the cure is Scripture. This will give God the opportunity to join in the conversation. Then she said "to reach out to God through meditation." So I tried.

I knew I needed to change my thought patterns and reprogram my mind in order for me to handle everything that was happening to me. I was trying to be aware of everything and everyone around me so my thought patterns were positive.

I really believe that those tinctures herbal extracts Dr. M had me on were really causing me more harm than I realized at the time.

I was finally able to leave the house; I was in so much pain from sitting and laying down that my back and hips were killing me. I made an appointment to go see Dr. S; he was very upset with what had been going on and told me to stop seeing Dr. M. But I didn't. Dr. S was great at nurturing his patients, encouraging me to stay focused on what was happening to me and to my body.

As time went on, I started noticing some really bizarre skin conditions. My skin on my chest, shoulders, breast, and stomach started to split or blister. They were nasty looking, itched and burned; I was very distraught over what was happening to my skin. I was due to see my family doctor, Dr. N, and he was shocked at what was happening to me and extremely angry with Dr. M. He also told me I needed to stop seeing Dr. M. He said, "I know you are in a situation with your health and with all the diseases you have that have come on aboard along the way, but I am seriously afraid of what other harm may come your way while seeing Dr. M!"

I continued on with Dr. M, trying to give him the benefit of the doubt, but I was sadly mistaken. When you have Lyme disease, it is very difficult to know the right thing or treatment protocol to use.

My dear, sweet, patient husband was just as distraught as I was; he wanted me to stop seeing Dr. M also. I was so embarrassed to even let my husband see my skin.

I started noticing my skin blistering and then splitting. I called Dr. M and asked if I could come to his office to show him what my skin was doing, and he said, "No, I want you to go to your family doctor and let him give you a diagnosis and then return to me and I'll treat it!"

I told Dr. M, "If you can't diagnose this skin condition, I have to stop seeing you."

When I decided to leave Dr. M, I had no idea what I was about to encounter with my health. I thought having Lyme disease, Rocky Mt. Spotted Fever, and all my other decaying health conditions was enough but then my life became unbearable!

After I left Dr. M, I started having bouts of cold body temperatures. I was froze all the time. I noticed a lump in my throat (neck); my nails, hair, and skin were dry and brittle; my weight started to climb; moody, low libido, fatigue, memory problems, confusion, can't stay focused, coughing, and stomach pain.

In January of 2006, my health problems continued on a downward spiral.

I went to a medical imaging office, where I was placed on a treadmill and had topographic images of my heart studied. After that I was sent to another imaging therapy where they did a Two-D-M-mode echocardiography was obtained with Doppler supplementation. The doctor informed me that one of my mitral valves wasn't closing tightly."

February 2, 2006 I ended up having a skin pathology on the base of my neck.

I ended up back in Dr. N's office with my skin eruptions and a rash. I had developed a cough, acute laryngitis, acute sinusitis, and an upper respiratory infection. Dr. N issued an antibiotic and an injection to keep the URI from turning into pneumonia and ordered bed rest!

March 30, 2006, I dislocated my left foot falling down the steps from upstairs bedroom in the hallway. Three days later my husband drove me to a local hospital, where I was treated for a fractured left foot. Dr. S wanted to have a look at X-rays and sent me to have an image run. He was trying to determine what caused this unfortunate event. I continually used the salt baths, resting the foot, icing the foot, wrapping in the bandage, walking with crutches, and continuing my back and leg therapies.

I went into Dr. S's office, and he decided to put me on some new natural medications to help me with my skin eruptions. Dr. S showed me a product called Silver Hydrosol; once again we were turning our attention to Silver as a primary immune support tool. Its use as a respected preservative, disinfectant, and regenerative agent dates back thousands of years. A hydrosol is defined as a colloid in which pure water is the medium. A colloid refers to a suspension of fine particles dispersed in a gas or liquid. It is a colloid of micro-fine silver particles dispersed in ultrapure water, free of any other ingredient or contaminant.[17]

In April I continued to see Dr. B, who was a podiatrist for my foot treatments.

In May I started to develop esophagus and stomach problems. Eating was becoming a serious problem as well as coughing, chest pains, stomach pains, itching, and skin eruptions. I was already following a nutritional diet when I was seeing Dr. S, and I was eating just fruits and vegetables, fish, chicken, lean pork, red meat on occasion, trying to stay away from sugar and cutting back on coffee. So I felt I was eating in a correct manner and being careful about staying away from carbohydrates.

Dr. N wanted me to see a specialist, and I conferred with Dr. S as well. I was soon sent to Dr. R, who was a gastroenterologist. I discussed the problems I was having, and he also noticed on my chart that I have Lyme disease, which I already knew was going to be a problem. The majority of medical doctors that I have been to "get an attitude" with me over my Lyme disease and want to dismiss it. But I have never backed down from them, and I don't let the doctors try to discourage me from finding the problems. The majority of doctors do not believe Lyme disease exists, they dismiss it. I feel that Lyme disease is very political. Infectious diseases are generally treated with antibiotics until patients are well, but some medical doctors follow guidelines from IDSA (Infectious disease society of America) using unchanged guidelines for Lyme designed to restrict diagnosis and to limit treatments beyond flawed guidelines. With delayed diagnosis, combined with limited treatment this is a recipe for chronic illness to set in. The mainstream medical community would rather treat each symptom separately that way there's more to profit from.

Yes, it is true that every test that I've had to endure, the test results come back negative and the usual culprit is from the underlying Lyme disease. Lyme disease is a complicated disease that wears many faces! Dr. R sent me for an Endoscopy, I went in as an out patient to a local hospital. My trusted friend, my mother-in-law, drove me, sat by my side reading a book while my test was being performed. The nurses' staff placed an IV drip with Ampicillin in my arm. This brought back horrible memories of what I went through seven years ago when I was finally diagnosed with the Lyme disease. I was terrified of the IV and started to hyperventilate, but I vowed that I wasn't going to give up and I lay there and prayed God would be with me throughout this test, and He was!

Then the nurse gave me an injection of Gentamyacin for sleep gazing, then Demerol. They took a biopsy of my intestine to determine why I was having such a difficult time with certain foods. They were looking for a disease called Celiac Disease—a disease that cannot tolerate wheat and gluten.

Seven days later the report came back, which meant I would have to go back to Dr. R's office to get the results.

He said, "The biopsy was clear. No Celiac Disease I told Dr. R about the elimination diet I was on and how much better I felt. Then he said, "You need to have a colonoscopy." I told him I needed to think about it.

On August 3, I went to Dr. S, and he put me on a detox program; his program was mild, and I was able to leave the house and not fear losing control of my bowels. I was even able to lose a few pounds!

I went back to Dr. S to start another new round of natural medications. This was a good group for energy and to help build the immune system. I know it sounds like a lot to take, but it's all natural medicines and nothing that will harm my internal body like the synthetic drugs that the mainstream medical community prescribes. One day I was outside working in my flowers and a bee stung me. My knee swelled up the size of my fist. I iced it and rubbed bag balm (antiseptic used on cow's udders) nice thought, huh? It took the swelling out so I was able to bend my knee.

When I get stung my skin turns a bright red as though I pressed myself with an iron. I was having a difficult time with my left foot, especially underneath the foot. I found it difficult to walk.

I made an appointment with a Dr. C, another podiatrist, for a follow up with my injured foot. He found that my left foot had a fracture on the top part of the foot. He decided to put me in a walking cast. Dr. C and I started a conversation about the Lyme disease and he felt that my bone structure and muscles were slowly deteriorating from the disease. Dr. C orders a TENS unit, bone stimulator to use at home. It's a hand-held computer; you wrap a Velcro attachment around your foot then add a gel to the pads and stick the pad on your foot (top of foot), program the machine for twenty minutes. You can't feel anything, but it's helping heal the fracture.

I'm trying to be a good patient and not so moody, but I'm just tired of what keeps happening to me. It's not getting easier; it seems as though there's always setbacks. I decided to write some poems again, asking God for his help and patience.

I have so many doubts
And fears every day.
Sometimes the pain
Just won't go away.
But I know you care
And I know you are there.
So please, Lord Jesus,
Just show me the way!
Loving and kind
Your words are divine
My life wouldn't be
Complete without You
Showing me the way.
I'm so thankful
That you still live today
Cause you've shown me the way.
What blessings you shower
On all of us each day.
When we come to you trusting
And lovingly obey.
Lord Jesus, your way
You're the only way
Goodness and mercy
You teach us to share
All the love you have given,
Gives us time to prepare
For the wonderful times
That we'll have with you up there
Because you have shown us,
Shown us the way!

This is how I've lasted as long as I have. I'm fortunate to still be alive! I know of many chronic Lyme disease patients who are not fairing as well and of others who have died. I know that God has given me abilities to reach out and help others who are not able to do for themselves; he's given me a voice, mind, two strong hands and the courage to stand up and fight for Lyme disease.

I'm having a difficult time sleeping. Dr. S performs a cranial adjustment on my head; I slept like a baby that night.

I've been using an antibiotic for my Lyme disease as a maintenance dose. My husband, of course, agrees with their diagnosis.

I have learned that with illness (and I'm not just talking about the Lyme disease) it's important to own a positive outlook. You also need to keep an open mind, sense of humor, and balance.

It's funny, but I never really had a great deal of faith in the beginning, and I was the last person you'd ever want to discuss Jesus with. I couldn't stand hearing about it. My sisters were a bunch of "Bible thumpers," always pushing me with their scriptures and so forth. Now look at me—I'm leaning toward God, read scriptures, and study the Bible. My older sister laughed the other day when she asked me to pray for her and I started to.

Now I depend on God to help me get through all of it. This one particular sister stepped in when I lost my oldest sister and we have come "full circle" again. I admire her strength and the great love she has for Jesus. My brothers and sisters are quite older than I am; being the youngest of eleven children, now there are only seven of us here today.

I was afraid of death, but I'm not anymore. It's not fearing death itself, it's the leaving part, leaving your loved ones behind and being an important part of their lives also not being able to watch them grow, especially the little ones. I know now that for the faithful, dying is as much a beginning as an end. It's just a gateway to heaven where there is no more pain and sickness. I have found strength in God, I shall prevail; I may be weak on the outside but God is providing me with strength on the inside. I'm standing up for what's right. I'm looking for a higher purpose. I pray for God's guidance; I want to uncover the source of Lyme disease's problems and take a plan of action!

Dr. C ordered another X-ray on my foot. He ordered the nurse to give me an injection (no steroids, please); steroids cause the Lyme disease too grow. He ordered me to start taking the walking cast off and to exercise the foot.

It's a new day I want to tell everyone how much God loves them and what He has done for me. I'm enjoying my surroundings, and the love of my family, life has a way of removing them quickly. Don't take anything for granted, you never know what's going to happen. Listen to the music that nature provides the beauty that surrounds us, lift up thy voice and tell him of your love, He will reward you, In His own time!

I told my granddaughter, Monet, "Reach Up, Little Child, Touch the sky, see how God Loves you and so do I, Don't be afraid, He's with you today, Just kneel on your knees and Pray, Pray, Pray!" She always shouts with joy when I make up poems or stories, even though she herself is only three years old she has my Lotus the Pug poem memorized.

I had another poem come to mind pertaining to the doctors who misdiagnosed me, it is as follows:

Lyme Ticks Will Make You Sick

Deer ticks in Ohio, No, No!
That's what the doctors say
Then what's this rash on me?
Just rub some cream on it; it
Will go away!
Well, it didn't as I can see
Now my head aches
My neck is stiff, now, Doc, will you agree?
There are deer ticks in Ohio
Don't you see?
You're just nervous, he'd say
Will run some tests another day
You'll see, there's nothing there
What's it going to take for these doctors to care?
Well, here I am
Been bit with a deer tick
Now I'm starting to feel very sick
As I continue to worsen
The doctor continues to disagree
Lyme disease in Ohio. No! That can't be!
It's hard on us, Doc, can't you see?
Our lives are so uncertain
I'm tired of my body always hurting.
Please, please won't you help us
So we can become antibiotic free and live our life the way God meant it too be!
Lyme in Ohio, oh no that can't be

Until you've been bit, Ohhh yes
You will see.
What I've been trying to say
Unless you get bit by a nasty deer tick
Will you finally agree, yes oh yes
There are Lyme ticks in Ohio and then
You will agree!

I love reading II Corinthians 4:8–10, 18. I was watching Joyce Meyer, and she was talking about how to defeat depression and being stuck in your life.

I love listening to her; she is a wonderful woman, and she herself has overcome many obstacles. She has prevailed, and now she's opening doors for others as I want to open doors for people who can't get the proper diagnosis.

Dr. N ordered another blood test; he was shocked when it came back. My cholesterol, triglycerides, HDL, and LDL were elevated but not by much. "What's going on here? What are you doing differently?" he asked me.

Dr. N was still concerned over my high CRP (coronary reactive protein). He also said my hemoglobin was a little elevated. He mentioned metabolic syndrome, toxins, and steroid overuse in my system. Then he made a comment about my Lyme disease, and I said, "Wait a minute, Doc? How about all thirteen doctors that I saw before I was finally diagnosed with these diseases? a All the medications, inflammatories, all the steroids that the previous doctors abused my body with." Dr. N also mentioned about my digestive problems he found in my blood tests, the gluten and wheat sensitivities that my body is unable to break down, he also found that I was lactose intolerant.

I was scheduled to see Dr. C to get an evaluation on my foot. I prayed that the tens unit (bone stimulator) is working and mending the fracture.

I went back to Dr. C for a checkup on my fractured foot, and he ordered me to go for physical therapy.

The therapist and his staff were all very knowledgeable instructors and were also compassionate about my physical therapy and were spellbound about all the health problems that I have. It was tough at times and the therapy was slow, but I knew I would be in for a long haul. That's how it is with Lyme disease, you can't get ahead of it; there is always some other health issue that arises. I went to physical therapy three times a week for a long time. My therapist would place my left foot in a whirlpool tub, and the hot swirling water would help to alleviate stiffness in my foot. Then the therapist would rotate my ankle and exercise the foot trying to regain strength and momentum.

Between my therapies and trying to babysit my granddaughter, Monet, my husband and I decided to go to New York City to spend Thanksgiving with our youngest daughter, Corinne. I was also in the process of trying to organize a support group again. I spoke to another Lyme disease friend and asked her if she would like to help me. So I wrote up an article for our local newspaper called "Tick-Talk" and asked her to place it in the health notes section of our paper.

So we contacted all of our Lyme disease friends we knew in our community and surrounding areas to ask others who would be interested in an evening or a day out. I was telephoned by a gentleman in PA who was very sick with Lyme disease and heard about what we were trying to put together. He said, "I have other diseases prior to the Lyme disease, and I've never felt as bad; it's a debilitating, devastating, painful, degrading experience. My heart just sank while I was on the phone with him because I understood everything he said.

My friend and I didn't receive many calls for a meeting. I told the doctors who I wanted to come and speak, one was a Lyme disease doctor and the other doctor was a ND. My Lyme disease doctor tried to tell me that "many Lyme disease victims are so frustrated with this disease they're afraid to get involved or too ill, tired, and unable to attend." So many of them feel as though the mainstream medical community, their own doctors, their families, their government has let them down and that going to a support group meeting is effortless. I soon found out that this was true; when I called many other Lyme disease victims, I didn't get a very nice response either. My friend who was helping me didn't have much luck. In fact, she herself bowed out from helping me because she was so sick and not interested in attending the support group meeting.

I discussed this with my naturopathic doctor who I was going to ask to speak at our support group meeting, and he was very disappointed over this also.

November 18, 2006

I asked Dr. C if I could go to New York City with my husband for Thanksgiving. He had given me a clean bill of health to go. I was out of the walking cast, but I still continued to use the tens unit for therapy. He said, "You need to rest the foot and use the machine for ten minutes a day, but just take it easy, please!"

We packed our truck and loaded up for NYC. I was looking forward in visiting Corinne; we hadn't seen her for six months. It was fun traveling once again, but I needed to stop driving; we gassed up the truck, stopped and ate some lunch.

We arrived in the concrete jungle, hot, tired, and ever so anxious to see her. My heart lifted when I saw her, and I walked up to her and gave her a big hug and kiss. It was wonderful to finally get to see my little baby again. She hugged her dad and everything was right with the world again. I forgot about everything I was experiencing—all the pain, the Lyme disease, everything, and it was an awesome feeling. I felt like a brand-new person! She helped us unload our truck; we brought her some food staples to stock her kitchen, also we brought most of the preparations for our Thanksgiving dinner in the big city.

We finished our first day out in the big city—visiting, laughing, and talking—and I decided I needed to sit down and rest. I placed my tens unit on my foot for my treatment for twenty minutes, and I couldn't wait to go to bed. I was exhausted! I believe from all the excitement, nervousness, anxious feelings of coming to NYC, being in the city with all of its hustle and bustle and seeing our daughter just wore me out, and I knew if I didn't get myself under control, it would be a rough week for me. I slept like a baby that night!

I was so excited about attending the Macy's Day Parade. We took our umbrellas with us, security was on every corner and in between the balloons could barely stay afloat from the wind and the rain. We didn't stay long. I was wiped out and wanted to return to the apartment; everyone else agreed. We stopped at Angela's Coffee Shop in her neighborhood and ate breakfast; then we came back up to the apartment to prepare our turkey. I went to lie down while the turkey was roasting, Dave and Corinne went for a walk.

I awoke from a great rest, and we all prepared for our Thanksgiving dinner.

I had my scheduled appointments running through my mind, couldn't wait to get home for a back treatment and Dr. S's office. Time flew while we were in NYC.

JANUARY 01, 2007

A lot took place after our trip in November of 2006 to NYC. I had another fracture in my left foot; the first one I had was a hairline fracture. This one now is split, so back in my big, black walking cast we go again.

In the meantime, I developed another respiratory infection. I went into see Dr. N, and he prescribed a Z pack—an antibiotic used to treat bacterial infections.

On January 11, I went back to Dr. J, my Lyme disease doctor, and we discussed my problems with the continuous infections of my respiratory system, and he decided to try me on a drug called Bicillin, 600,000 units (injection). This drug is to be administered by a nurse or a doctor, injected into a large muscle—the butt muscle!

The antibiotics work best when the amount of medicine in your body is kept at a constant level. This is done by scheduling the dosage at evenly spaced intervals. If more than one dose is required, make sure you do not miss any doses. The number of doses depends on the type of injection. Continue receiving this medication until the fully prescribed treatment program is finished or if symptoms disappear after a few days. Stopping this medication too early may allow bacteria to continue to grow, resulting in a relapse of the infection. (This is how my Lyme disease doctor, Dr. J, explained it.)

This drug may cause mild diarrhea, upset stomach, nausea, vomiting, or irritation at the injection site.

I continued having an infection in my lungs once again. Dr. N ended up putting me on decongestants and a cough syrup. My husband kept worrying about this scenario of what I've had to go through and said it reminded him of what I experienced ten years prior when I found out I had Lyme disease. "Yes, it is true, dear. It's a terrible reminder of what I've had to deal with, and I'm not looking forward to what I may experience now with this infection in my lungs." These infections are always a great concern that they could turn into pneumonia.

Dr. J put me on the Bicillin for five weeks to see how I'd react, hopefully, to slow the Lyme down, help heal my bones, and make everything else feel better.

We have no timelines to when to stop using the antibiotics; the Lyme doctor isn't able to determine how long it takes. There are signs and everyone reacts differently. Some people have been on antibiotics for five years and longer, are no longer using them and are doing fine. Then there are others who can't be off of the drug for very long, and I have fallen into this category. I manage about two years off of the drugs; then I develop respiratory complications and that's when I know I'd better be heading back to my Lyme disease doctor and start the drug again.

There is no 100 percent positive test for Lyme disease. If a patient doesn't see a Lyme literate doctor to do a PCR test (to determine or a western blot, antibody assay), Lyme antibodies must be present for a positive result. If the patient was using steroids, Advil, Motrin, or other anti-inflammatory or antibiotics, this could result a false-negative report[18].

Healing with Lyme disease is a lifelong journey, and I pray that it won't be a final destination! I went into my family doctor's office for an injection because my nurse friend wasn't available yet to give me the shot. The nurse at Dr. N's office was a little rough, and it really hurt that time. I had been running a low-grade fever and headache was forming from the injection. Carrie, our oldest daughter, came down and tried to give me the injection, but she was very nervous about doing so, so my neighbor came down and gave it to me. It was so slick and fast, I never even felt the needle going in, just a bit of burning from the drug flowing into my system.

I really feel the weight piling on; when I look at myself in the mirror, I don't recognize that person anymore. This disease has changed me drastically in so many way—it's changed my appearance, muddies my thinking; I'm much quieter than I use to be, I don't call my siblings or friends on the telephone, I keep to myself, I don't go out in public too often, only to do things that need to be addressed. Then I return home, to my sanctuary.

I went to see Dr. S for a back treatment and a treatment on my left wrist. I have developed tendonitis and I am wearing a brace on it!

JANUARY 30

Put in another bad night, violent dreams, confusing thoughts. I'm not watching Monet anymore. I had her here one day a week, but she's in daycare and with that being said, she catches colds and flu; then it becomes a concern that I may catch the germs. So I had to stop watching her for the winter and concentrate on my wellness.

My left hand is sore; my body is falling apart piece by piece, seems as though there's an awful lot of misfortunes happening with my body right now. I dream of spring and how I want to put in a raised bed garden and pray that I can work in my flowerbeds. I guess that is what keeps me going; this gives me hope and reassurance. I'm sitting here in my recliner with my left foot propped up, my left hand on ice, and I know it is for my own good. Jesus knows our pain and suffering.

My oldest sister who has now passed away would always tell me, "Jesus knows your pain, for He is the one who laid down His life for me and you; to trust in Him is difficult to do for many, but for me, I have learned through all my hardships to lean on Him! No one in your life can help you through these difficulties that life can burden you with; you need to lean on Jesus's strengths. Not even your spouse, children, or family can help you, but Jesus can and He does! I'm amazed at how I've turned my problems over to Jesus, how I depend on His love and guidance. When I think about what my life without Jesus could have been, I'm thankful now to have been given the opportunity to depend on Him, and I know in my heart, this was His plan for me all along!

We all get caught up in our own problems and misgivings. We have so much to be grateful for, and yet we take so much for granted. Everyone on this planet has had and does share difficulties in their own lives; some are far more worse than others, there's so much pain and suffering in many lives—fear and illness. But if we all could just take a deep look at ourselves inside and truly find what is really important and not sweat the small stuff, life could be easier for all of us. We humans put ourselves through so much hurt and aggravation that it's difficult to realize life can be easier if we just slow down and take life one day at a time. We need to be more like children, carefree, loving, funny, playful, and just be ourselves. Enjoy each day, don't rush through life, live in the moment!

I went back to Dr. S for another back and foot treatment on August 31, 2006. I went to therapy for the foot (hot water therapy), stretching the foot to regain strength in it. I went to see Dr. C about the foot, X-rays were given. He revealed, "Your bones are healing nicely and filling in like they are supposed to." He wanted to keep me in the walking cast for another two weeks. He also fitted me with an ankle brace to wear inside my shoes around the house for three hours at a time, then back into the walking cast. I promised Dr. C that I wouldn't take anymore trips where walking was a requirement. He was happy too hear that! He also felt that the injection I was getting was helping with the bones mending. I did not have nearly the pain and tenderness in that foot!

Dr. C said, "I want you to go to a local sporting goods store and buy a hiking boot; wear your orthotics in the boots.

My dear, sweet husband has a hard time understanding why I'm not chipper and laughing at times.

He cleaned off the table for me and put the food away while I just sat and stared out the window. I spotted two deer and five more sitting alongside our pond huddled together just minding their own business. I guess they feel safer here close by. Dave feels that the deer are coming closer because of the coyotes out in the field. At night you can hear them yelping, and I'm sure the deer come here to find security and safety. So with the growing deer population, wild coyotes are looking for some form of food source. Our pets and our families are in danger of what lurks on these animals bodies. I know all too well what ticks can carry, dangerous insects they are!

February 3, 2006—I had another rough night, wrist, left hip aches and hurts, woke up with a headache. My husband asked me to ride along with him to pick up some parts, and we'll stop to get breakfast. I was excited for Monet to come over so we could work on Valentine crafts; she helps to take my mind off of everything when she comes over.

I had Monet today, and we played and worked on our crafts. She stayed with me for a while longer today; her parents had a(n) episode happen that required medical attention. By the end of the day, I was pooped. So Poppy (that's what Monet calls her grampa), cleaned up the crafts and the toys while the three of us managed to put some food on the table. It was a very emotional day for me. My son-in-law had his foot wrapped around the shaft of a wood splitter, and my husband had to untangle his foot; fortunately, he wasn't hurt severely. But it made me terribly anxious and exhausted for him.

I offered to drive my son-in-law to pick up Monet at the sitter's house. He was on crutches and I in my walking cast; we sure looked funny to the babysitter. Monet helped me walk out to the truck, and Troy managed to get into the truck himself. Thank goodness the cast is on my left foot so at least I can drive.

I feel more energized but can't say that my left wrist is any better. Dr. S did a treatment on my wrist and told me to start drinking Noni Juice, known to help with inflammation. I slept without my cast on, and my foot even feels better. I'm actually starting to feel really good again.

I wrote another poem.

THE WINTER SNOW

Outside it's cold
The snow is falling.
Inside it's warm
Our hearts are calling.
The days seem long
The months creep so slowly.
Outside the snow is falling
Another winter is gone.
Tucked away inside the snow
Are all the creatures big and small
Who find it nice and sweet
To rest and keep warm
To enjoy their winter and be free from harm.
Inside our hearts are warm
Our hands, our minds
Rest comes easy for some
For winter to be over
Tucked away for another year.

I just keep writing my thoughts down; it keeps me from going insane. It certainly has been a long winter and cold too. Resting is easy, patience is rough, but I try. I sure hope spring will arrive soon and that I will be able to participate and enjoy my surroundings free of wrist guards and walking casts.

It was another struggle for sleep. I heard my husband coughing. I woke up and he wasn't in bed beside me. I was concerned for him. At 6:00 a.m. I woke up, put my walking cast back on, and came hobbling downstairs to fix breakfast for my husband. I looked outside and there were two does right by the garage door and one doe by my butterfly bush. I've got to do something to discourage these animals from coming to close to my house. TICKS, TICKS, TICKS—not a good thing! I have so much pain in my fingers and hand I find it difficult to hold a pen in my hand or hold the receiver of the phone. I called and cancelled my appointment with Dr. J; the weather is unpredictable, and I'm afraid to drive myself over there to his office.

FEBRUARY 14, 2006

Happy Valentine's Day, everyone! I was taking a shower, drying off and examining my skin. It's awful looking—so many abrasions, scars; it's horrible. This bothers me more than my husband; I'm going to have to use some type of concealer or something to cover my skin. I would never wear a bathing suit or even a short-sleeve top anymore because of how awful my skin looks. God bless my husband; he offered to take me up to a lodge for the weekend as a pick-me-up for Valentine's Day, but I refused. They have a beautiful indoor pool, and I love to swim and so does my husband, but it would be mortifying to me to put on a swimsuit.

FEBRUARY 15

I cancelled my Lyme disease doctor's appointment because I wasn't feeling well. I was too nervous and anxious to drive to his office, so he sent me a script for lab work and a three-week RX for the Bicillin injection pack. I worked on the computer, entering some items and checked my emails. I received an e-mail from a French doctor who has two Lyme disease patients in his hospital, one with meningitis and the other with Lyme disease; they both have inflammation in their back and their joints! I want to email him and tell him I also suffer with Lyme disease and see if he has any other treatment protocols that possibly I could try. I am always looking and researching other avenues and educating myself for new therapies, new medications, whatever I can find. I look and wait.

I drove over to my natural foods store for more Noni Juice. I can't begin to tell you how this juice has helped me, especially my left wrist where the pain was so severe. I haven't worn my wrist guard for one whole week, and I'm not experiencing the sharp, dull pain that I usually have with it. I'm so blessed to have Dr. S, he really knows his stuff!

I'm sitting here listening to my Native American Indian CD and feeling all is well. It's my lucky day injection day, and my husband will be administering it. I know he's nervous about doing this.

FEBRUARY 20

I'm fasting for a blood test. I went for labs and picked up my medications. I'm still achy and hurt all over. I went to see Dr. S for a back treatment and to order vitamins and supplements. Everything that I am using from him is helping, so I need to stay on them. I went in to see Dr. N for my Lyme Titer, IMG, and IGG tests for Lyme to see if the injection is slowing the Lyme down. I also went to see Dr. C; he's happy with my foot. He also wants me to start therapy again.

FEBRUARY 22

I'm writing again little poems, little notes, gestures, whatever it takes to keep my mind off of everything. We all need a guardian angel, and my little angel is Monet; she amazes me and makes me laugh and has an insatiable smile that melts my heart.

ANGELS

There are angels among us now.
Look up and see them; they're everywhere
In your heart, your mind
We don't know how
But they're always there
Just waiting for you.
Don't be afraid, they say
We'll be with them soon, someday
So laugh, love, and play
The angels are among us tomorrow and today!

You never know when you speak to a stranger if they were put here for a reason, to protect us or just watch over us. But whatever the reason is, there's always an explanation. We are not to be afraid to suffer because God is watching over us and with us. He is always there waiting for us to ask for His help. Having Lyme disease has taught me to walk in faith and to know God's love. It has taught me humility and has given me an inner strength that I didn't know I possessed. I'm trying to encourage my husband to take his mother who's seventy-five years old and go to NYC to visit Corinne.

I slept good but woke up with a headache again; it's either from the cheese I ate or the wine I had. I usually get a sore throat from eating cheese and a headache as well.

Sleeping was tough I hurt all over; my body ached, and I couldn't get comfortable no matter what, and I was coughing a great deal. I'm really going to have to watch my eating patterns—no more cheese, dairy, milk, butter, sugar, gluten, wheat, etc. I need to change my eating habits to only fruits, veggies, and a little meat.

My hubby and I are going out to buy me a pair of hiking boots.

My therapy class is today and things are going well for me! My niece is coming to clean for me also and that's great too. She's a big help for me in more ways than I can ever tell her.

MARCH 8

It's Dave's and my evening out to see The Blue Man Group. I also had to make a trip over to my Lyme disease doctor. He told me, "Your labs are showing that the Lyme disease is very active, and I need to stay on the injection." He also told me, "You don't have any new infections from the Lyme disease, but the RMSF spots on your shins are active, that's why they burn and itch to the point of bleeding."

I have to be so careful when I shave my legs because the spots on my legs from the RMSF bleed. My husband said, "Please wash that towel with all the blood on it because if you would happen to die in the middle of the night, I don't want anyone to think I had something to do with your departure." I just laughed and threw it in the washer for him.

Dr. J also told me, "You keep that positive energy you have." But he also told me not to multi-task, do one thing at a time, finish, then go to the next thing, keep resting, stay interested in things you are doing, keep laughing, keep writing, sailboat season will be coming soon and enjoy Monet. I hesitated telling my husband that Dr. J wanted me to stay on the drug for six more weeks, but I knew he needed to know since he was the one giving the injections to me.

I have terrible nightmares, horrible things I dream of, and I don't know how I can think such nasty things. It has to be from the drug, or am I delusional? I wandered around the house for a while trying to get sleepy and to put nasty thoughts out of my mind.

It was another quiet day, trying to stay off of my left foot. I do not need this bone to fracture again. I'm tired and the injection is really throwing me for a loop! I know the stress in my life is bad right now, not a good substance when fighting Lyme disease. Dr. S put me on potassium drops to use to help dry up the sinuses. I will monitor this cold, and if I need to I will go and see my family doctor. I can't take the chance of getting pneumonia! Dr. S is aware of my difficulties I have with my health and doesn't interfere. My immune system seems to be turning on me the weather is damp and rainy, and I proceeded to cancel therapy for the rest of the week. I need to stay home in quiet, rest and keep warm.

APRIL 3

I went to Dr. S for a laser treatment on my lungs; it's amazing and it is still working for me.

I cancelled appointment with Dr. J. I went back to bed too weak and too tired.

APRIL 10

I woke up disgusted. I need to be doing my therapy. I just don't want to go, but I pushed myself over there and worked out for forty-five minutes, and I was wiped out. I came home to rest, try and fix dinner, woke up head was full and congested, hurt all over all the way down to my feet.

APRIL 12

I woke up refreshed slept pretty good for a change. I ordered some lavender oil to spray on my pillow at night; this is suppose to invoke calmness and sleep. I can't believe it actually works! I have to get dressed and go over to the Lyme disease doctor, and I invited my dear friend Carole to ride along with me. She has been the sweetest friend, but I have to remember she has many health problems as well, and she continues to keep on going, being involved, and I appreciate her so much for that.

I told Dr. J about the injections and how they are starting to affect the left side of my body. He wants me to stay on the injections for a while longer. Dr. J called Dr. N and told him, "I want Janet to start strength and balance training at her therapy." Dr. N called my therapist to follow up the order from Dr. J.

I woke up with a terrible headache, but I went to my therapy. He decides to see just how much of a work out I can withstand. I do seem to have more stamina and energy when I'm exercising. My brother stopped over, and when he looked at my counter he asked, "Do you take all those pills?" I said, "Yes, because they all work!" He shook his head in amazement!

I try to remain positive. God will provide. God will answer in His own time, not when I want Him to!

I had appointment with Dr. C to determine how foot is recovering, pressed and twisted foot, keep the brace on it, start walking one mile a day up and down your driveway at least five times.

I went to my therapy class; my left knee is causing trouble again and my lower back is hurting as well.

Sleep was better although my legs cramped up considerably, coughing, sore throat and congested. There's a constant pain in the left side of my throat, not sore, but difficulty with swallowing. I continued to walk my mile; my body is hurting me especially the left side; my left knee is hurting and the left side of my throat is painful.

I am so sick and tired of this disease and yes, I'm ticked off!

I went to Dr. S so he could do a back treatment and adjust my left knee for me.

My knee has a tendency to pop out of place, so Dr. S put it back in place for me.

I was down on the Internet on my Lyme disease sites, and I saw a major breakthrough for chronic Lyme disease victims. Dr. Fallon in New York and other Lyme disease associations have opened a research center at Columbia University for Lyme disease and other tick-borne diseases on April 30. This is a massive breakthrough for all chronic Lyme disease. Now the whole world needs too hear about this progress. A notable author, Amy Tan, who also suffers with Lyme disease, calls it, "A Center for Hope" for all Lyme disease victims. (Dr. Fallon Research Center for Chronic Lyme disease in New York)

Then there's the old adage when people come up to you and say, "You don't look sick, you look good." It brings me to what a young person who died with Lyme disease would say to her mother: "Mom, it is bad enough to be sick and have Lyme disease, but it is worse to have to keep proving it over and over again." This was from a book dedicated to a young woman who gallantly fought her way through Lyme disease. The book is called *Twice An Angel: Living and Dying with Lyme Disease.*[19]

This is why I have chosen to only present myself to my own family members and most importantly to all the other Lyme disease victims and families who themselves are constantly fighting to keep going; we can't give up this fight, and we must prevail and be heard.

I'm tired of explaining myself to others who have no idea what living with chronic Lyme disease is like on a constant basis. I am trying to stay clear of the chatter that goes on in families. I don't need the stress of it all. I went to Casal's Spa & Salon to get facials, my hair colored, and styled. They served a part in my recovery efforts because it made me feel better about myself even if it only lasted for two or three days. I felt like I could handle life with a little more ease.

I've noticed my hair is thinning. I wonder if I need to ask Dr. N to check me for sugar or my thyroid. But I hesitate to do it because nine times out of ten I have tests run on me and they always come back negative and it's always the same culprit—the Lyme disease.

I've been trying to incorporate fruit into my diet and stay away from dairy products. This is proving difficult because I love cheese and to think I can't eat this anymore is frustrating. I'm congested, and it's either from the Maca (Pine Bark) or the Cat's Claw that I'm using for the Lyme. Pine trees is one of the big allergies I have, and I have them growing in my yard. I have to be careful to not let them brush up against my arms; I break out in hives and then I become itchy all over.

I made a decision to drop down from three days of therapy to just two days. It's taken a toll on me between Dr. S allergy treatments, back manipulations, and going in for my labs, I can't sustain this schedule.

April 12, 2007 It was my day to see Dr. J, and Carole rode along with me again. This friend has taught me so much about life and living; she has taught me to depend on God's love and patience. But one thing she has taught me the most is how to pray and not be embarrassed to do it. I don't understand why this is so difficult for me.

What is it that I'm so afraid of? Showing my vulnerability, my emotions, afraid of what other's might think? She's taught me to be myself and to not let others make me feel small and indifferent. I love her for that! She has tackled many health conditions herself; cancer has touched her life also, and she is still today fighting just like me.

Dr. J was delighted to see I'd lost eight pounds and that I was doing therapy twice a week, but he was a bit concerned about my blood work. So I had to fast again. He's watching my liver enzymes, and I'm thankful for that.

I fasted throughout the night, and I went in for my labs and was anxious to get my results. I ended up driving to the mall to have my frames on my glasses replaced. I developed an allergy to nickel so they were replacing them with titanium. I came home to rest. I don't know if I have any blood left in my body after all the lab work I just went through. My arms look(ed)s like a pincushion, and I bruise so easily now. The lab technicians have a difficult time drawing blood from me. My veins are so shallow that sometimes they place the needle on the top of my hands. The technicians do not like to go there, but sometimes they have no choice.

When I was resting I picked up my book *Time out for the Spirit* and was reading prayers for a family member who is going through a difficult time. It always seems to happen when our lives are so busy and full, someone seems to become ill or hurt; and although it can be a burden, it also can be a blessing. When I have my visions, I see my friend sitting on the bench where the light is so intense; it's awesome and inspiring. The colors are so rich and warm then I can hear her talking, but I can't see her.

June 7, 2007—My husband and I celebrated our 33rd anniversary. That's a long time with the same two people, but I'm just grateful to still be alive and able to cope with all of this.

I went to Dr. S to have my back manipulated and have him adjust my left knee. I had to show him my chest where I was breaking out with another lesion.

I've tried to keep positive people around me. My emotional well-being is crucial when you've been diagnosed with Lyme disease. I am genetically prone to fear or lack of involvement. I have negative feelings at times with stress, anxiety, and anger, and this can lower your immunity and cause hormonal shifts. It's important to keep tabs on other Lyme friends. This result means to avoid people who exhaust me or depress me. I believe that many in my family do not fully understand what it is like to have Lyme disease, and I'm not going to explain it to them anymore.

I went back to Dr. S for a back and knee treatment, trying to take it easy after my initial treatments. I placed an ice pack on my lower back and stayed in the house and decided the plants would have to do without me today.

I went back to Dr. S, and he tested my left knee. I managed to get to therapy, and my therapist agreed with Dr. S. My therapist placed me on a low-maintenance program until my X-rays came back. The X-rays showed that my knee wasn't in place, the knee is off to the side and the cartilage was torn. So I was in a knee brace for six weeks and using Synovial Fluid for joints.

It was another trip to my Lyme disease doctor and I took Carole along with me to give her a treat. Dr. J agreed with Dr. S that wearing the walking cast on my left foot for eight months had caused an imbalance in my body structure. We discussed all the problems I was having, and he wanted me to stay on the injections for one more month.

I slept good for a change but felt like I could have fallen back to sleep for a while longer, but I was planning on babysitting Monet for a while. I went to my therapy class, and my therapist studied my X-rays. He taped my knee and leg, rewrapped with the brace, and gave me exercises to do for over the weekend. I had a pretty good workout. I did a few cardiovascular exercises, and I can't believe how much more energy I am developing. Plus, I'm finally losing some weight.

I was watching a show one day on my religious network about how the prince is coming and how we need God in our lives now more than ever. There isn't mentioned much about God on TV or the papers; Sunday is just becoming another day for me, and I don't like it! I need to find a church home for myself. I should be studying God's words more than I do, praying for my soul and my family's as well. I want to find a church family so I can have peace and a place to worship with others who have their own issues. That way I can take Monet with me so she and I can find inner strength and contentment with knowing God and how much He loves us.

My husband heard on the news that President George Bush had Lyme disease and was treated for it. I wanted to e-mail him and see who he went to and what course of treatment he received or ask how long he went without a proper diagnosis.

The lesions are sore on my left upper breast but are healing some. Dr. S is trying to help me with all of this. I'm better but still have a long road ahead of me.

I say thumbs up to this wonderful doctor who has helped me reach my potential to make better health choices instead of relying on the medical doctors and getting the symptoms treated and not the real cause. Dr. S has taught me to think for myself, and I've learned how to talk to other doctors about my best interest as their patient. I'm very upfront with all my doctors, and they know it!

Dr. S mentioned that my adrenal system is faltering. This means my aging process will slow down, and I won't go as fast, which is good in a way. He says, "Chronic diseases can keep you from having heart attacks, strokes, or dementia."

I started my AF Beta Food first before I detox; my diet won't really change much because I'm eating fruits and vegetables, salads, chicken, turkey, and fish. While detoxing, eating red meat is not a good idea. I will be increasing my fluid intake and making slushies while consuming a great amount of water.

I told Carrie about my visit to Dr. J and my decision to stop using the drug for a while. She was delighted since she's not too keen on using antibiotics.

I slept pretty well last night; I prayed for my family like I do every night and prayed for strength to endure this battle. It was a busy day. I had my therapy class and worked out with my therapist. He told me, "You look like wonder woman pumping iron over there." I told him I was planning on getting nice and strong so I could go and beat up the doctors who misdiagnosed me.

The pain continues, I cancelled Dr. S's appointment. I'm just too tired to go, I find it's easier to just sit in my recliner; my body doesn't hurt as much if I stay still.

It was always great when I detoxed because I would lose weight easily, and I felt so much better after doing this. My liver, kidneys, and spleen are so overloaded with toxins in my system, I will do everything in my power to get this under control. Dr. S would reassure me, "It's not going to be an overnight fix." I need to try and stay off the injection for the Lyme disease as long as possible. While at Dr. S's, he strapped me in my knee brace again, and I came home.

Sleeping was rough again, my hands were numb, right hip hurt, don't feel well and my mind frame is off. I keep having nightmares, stemming from my fear of dying. Other dreams I have I can't remember, and some dreams I've blocked from my memory. But I do have a dream that I really am enlightened with; it's the one with my oldest sister, Marg, who died from cancer. I was walking down this long road, and I could see this glistening bright light from afar; and as I approached the area where the light was shining ever so brightly, I saw a park bench, and my sister was standing there. We hugged each other and laughed; then we sat down on the bench. She was beautiful, healthy, and happy, and we talked for hours. Then she said, "It's time for you to go back."

I said, "No, I want to stay here with you."

"Nope," she said, "it's not your time yet. Soon you can come be with me!" So as I started to walk away, I turned to look at her and she was gone! To me this is very comforting. I once was terrified, but now I'm thrilled at the prospect of dreaming and seeing them again.

I know in my heart that God has carried me through this, and I continue to do what I have to in order to keep going and getting better. "He is my Lamp, my guiding light. I'm like a small sailboat blowing in the harsh winds on the sea, being tossed about but never losing sight of the land ahead of me, where my God will be reaching out to me, calming the rugged seas and ever a soft blowing wind, He will guide me safely to shore!" As an example: When I am out sailing with my husband David I sometimes panic when the wind really picks up and the sailboat flies through the water. I look up into the sky and there is God watching over us reassuring me that everything will be fine, and it always is!

I went to my therapy to see Dr. S. It's funny, in his office all the other patients that come to see him with all their health issues; we have all become like one big family.

I slept really good again. I made a pot of herbal tea and made my breakfast for my better half, and I continued to detox. I went to therapy class and really had a good workout. I increased my reps by ten more; I was up to forty sets. My therapist told me, "The color in your face is improving, and you are really doing well with your exercises."

I called the Lyme disease doctor and told him about me not feeling well and my situation, and he told me, "The problem is from being off the injections because the injections masked the pain you were having." Now that I have been off the injection, I am starting to feel lousy and very nauseated.

I went to Dr. S for a treatment; he did acupressure and informed me of tests that I had pertaining to my liver, gallbladder, and stomach that were showing signs of weakness. I told him, "That's understandable when you consider all the drugs and antibiotics that I consumed over eleven years."

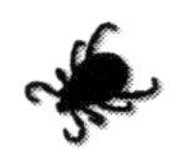

Hope on the Horizon

Dr. S showed me an article on Lyme disease and some new treatments that he's going to find out about for me and possibly we will experiment to see if we can kill off the cysts. Dr. S explained to me about biofilms that surround the Lyme disease bacteria, here it is: Biofilms are a sort of two edge sword. The cause of the biofilm is the body's response to an infecting organism, however this also prevents the destruction of said organism by antibiotics or antimicrobials. You see the body deposits fibrin so that the organism will be inhibited from being very mobile. If they are less mobile they can't do as much damage. Now here is the other side of the sword. The fibrin combines with heavy metals creating a barrier called a biofilm. This reduces or prevents antibiotics or anti-microbials from getting to the organism. Unless you break down this protective barrier you can't kill the Lyme. This is where my doctor, Dr. S's nutritional program comes into effect. First product is Nattokinase; it cleans the fibrin or breaks it down. The next step is to add an antimicrobial, like Argentyn 23, and the third product is a heavy metal chelator to remove these from the body as they are released from the biofilm. This program is individualized and should be supervised by a qualified physician. The dosage will gradually be increased wherein the program becomes effective. IF you don't do it right, It does not work. However, if you do it right you will be successful getting to the Lyme, and you will see wonderful results. What happens with Lyme disease is there are cysts that form off of the bacteria you get from the tick; it creates a cyst or a cocoon, and the drug is suppose to kill off the bacteria.

It really becomes overwhelming when you stop and think about what this tiny insect has and is doing to my body. If you concentrate on it, this can really be damaging to your mind. In all actuality, I'm terrified of the vision that I sometimes get thinking about this situation. I have horrible visions in my sleep of waking up and turning into a giant blood sucking tick, and everyone runs away from me screaming for their own life.

Monet didn't come to stay with me today because her parents were taking her to her pediatrician. Monet has a bite mark on her leg, bull's eye-shaped object. I told them make sure the doctor understands Lyme disease and to test for it. If it is Lyme disease, it can be detected and then be treated soon with a short course of antibiotics.

Carrie called and said the doctor thinks it's just a spider bite. I said, "Please keep an eye on this. If the bite mark should spread or Monet starts having bouts with other health problems, get her back into the doctor's office."

I was relieved to see Monet's leg was healing and the bite was nearly gone. Thank you, Jesus!

It was another night from beyond. I had a total of four hours sleep, coughing, but my throat feels so much better. My family and friends are calling me, but I don't answer the phone. I want so badly to just go to sleep; sometimes I want to sleep permanently. This disease is so aggravating, I can truly understand why some Lyme disease patients have taken their own lives. But then I stop and pray to God to help me stay focused on all of this that I'm living with, and He makes me realize not to give up hope!

I came downstairs to research on the Internet and found a product called Neem Oil; it's a natural form of cortisone from the evergreen tree, good for psoriasis, eczema that itchy complication. The smell isn't too pleasant, but it does seem to help. Another product I found was White Willow, a natural form of aspirin good for arthritis pain. Then I came across another product known as Eucalyptus Oil used for chronic sinus, ear infections, and bronchial. Put four drops of oil in a hot, steamy water-filled bowl, cover your head with a towel, lean over the bowl, and breathe in the steam. Then I found another one called Slippery Elm; this was used for coughs and congestion.

I went to my therapist, and he placed me in traction. I was amazed at how it made my back feel. It opens up the nerves so they're not pinched and opens up the discs. It looked like a device used in Medieval Times for torture, like a stretching machine. He strapped me on that table, and it holds you while the machine slowly stretches you, but I noticed a difference. I was a bit sore afterwards, so I iced my back when I came home.

I received a copy of *Woman's Day,* and there was an article about doctors' mistakes and misdiagnosis of diseases, and nothing was mentioned about Lyme disease. So I called their office, left my name and phone number, and told them I'd like to send in a short letter about Lyme disease. But I never got a response.

I went to Dr. S and had him look at these skin eruptions; we did an allergy treatment on them. Dr. S thought I should let my family doctor take a look also. When I arrived at Dr. L's office he had an intern from Ohio State University who came in first to examine me. I told him I had chronic Lyme disease; we talked about it, and he was very aware about Lyme disease and how the disease works. The intern suggested that I may have Lupus. Dr. L would need to run blood tests so we could try and decide what the spots were. I was so itchy in the night. I woke up bleeding from the spots.

I had an appointment with a specialist, Dr. RB; I went and discussed the homeopathic physician that I had seen when all these lesions started to appear. I told him he was "detoxing" me, and Dr. RB said, "I'm sorry, but I have to agree with Dr. S That the doctor you were seeing was toxifying your system." He then gave me Zrytec for the itching, steroid cream to alleviate the pain and the soreness and covered it with a bandage. He asked me to wait three weeks and then sent me for blood work after the skin heals.

I slept very well. The bandage doesn't seem too stay on my skin too well; the steroid cream and the zyrtec seemed to be helping. I had Monet today, so we made cut-out sugar cookies for Halloween and played.

I went to Dr. S. He wasn't overly amused with Dr. RB. He said, "I have other patients who see him, and they weren't too happy with his attitude."

I was sitting here talking to my other sister, and I told her about a quote I heard from Ellen Corby, Gramma on the Walton's: Things don't always come easy in this life. Most everything is hard work and prayers, but sometimes you've just got to know the bad things in life and just go on. That's the way of growing and being the best you can be.

This whole journey I've been through for twelve long years has been an education full of trust and distrust against our mainstream medical community and knowing when and how to let go and to just keep fighting my way through it all.

I went to see my foot doctor, Dr. C, and he examined my left foot and noticed a wart on my right foot. He froze the wart on my foot and put an antiseptic over it. He also made it clear to me that I was to wear shoes in the house all the time.

Dr. L called and said, "The rheumatoid panel is normal." It was my big day to meet with Dr. Y; he performed endoscopies and colonoscopies right there in his office. I sat in the waiting room and met some interesting people. Another patient in his office told me her sister in Staten Island, New York, has Lyme disease, and she said she's extremely ill with it. One thing led to the next, and I told her I had Lyme disease also. So we talked and exchanged phone numbers.

I finally met Dr. W, an associate of Dr. Y's. We sat down and discussed my health problems, and then he wanted to see my skin. He was shocked at what he was looking at and became very upset with Dr. RB. He ordered blood work, gluten panels, cell studies, colonoscopy, mammograms, and all my medical records to be released.

I slept well throughout the night, but I knew I had an appointment with Dr. RB to go over his reports with me. He performed a punch biopsy; this was a skin biopsy procedure in which a sample of skin tissue is removed, processed, and examined under a microscope. He's sending two grafts to two different locations, and then he proceeded to stitch me up. When I was out in the parking lot in my truck getting ready to leave, I felt like my blouse was wet, and when I unbuttoned my blouse, I was drenched with blood. I sat there holding the bandage and pressing on my incision when I had to call for assistance to have someone come out to help me back into the doctor's office. A nurse came out and helped me back into the doctor's room. I nearly passed out while the nurse was trying to get me into the room. Another patient was standing there and started to scream! I lay down on the table, and the doctor had to clean the biopsy and then had to stitch the incision over. My blood pressure dropped down to 90/70 they made me lay there for quite a while; they wanted someone to come and get me. I rested there for a short while and then I drove myself home. I called them when I arrived safely home. I applied pressure that the nurse instructed me to do, and I rested. The doctor also sent home creams to use on the incision.

Dr. L called and said, "The rheumatoid panel, gout, rheumatoid arthritis, lupus are all negative; the sedimentary rate is extremely high in the muscles, and your joints are full of inflammation." I was relieved that I didn't have Lupus, but as far as the sedimentary rate and the inflammation, this was not new to me. I already knew that the Lyme disease was the culprit behind everything.

I woke up at four o'clock in the morning congested and coughing, praying that I was not coming down with the flu.

My husband was concerned about my breathing. He knows all too well how Lyme disease works and the problems that it causes.

Dr. L called me in a z pack (zithromyacin). The doctor's are insisting I stop watching Monet. I called and asked Carrie if Monet could start going to daycare on my day that I was watching her. I felt bad about doing that, but I had no control over my health.

I called my other Lyme friend to check on her; she was struggling with this darn disease too. She had all kinds of gastrointestinal troubles and pain; we talked, we laughed, we prayed for each other. I'm so afraid I'll end up with pneumonia; sometimes I wonder how much longer I really have. I need to hang on; I have too much living to do yet, and I'm not ready to give up!

February of 2007 Dr. S went to a conference in Columbus, Ohio, over the weekend, and they spoke about Lyme disease. They have some new approaches on treating and killing off the burgforferi (bacteria), cells, macrophages and by using these natural products, it deletes the bacteria inside the cell structures. I told him to please order the products so I could start on this program.

I need to schedule with Dr. S and do a nutritional assessment by me bringing in all the vitamins and supplements that I use on a constant basis. I would like to watch the CD on how this program works. Dr. S said the conference should have been called Janet's Lyme Conference because everything they discussed hit me right on the nail!

I can't believe how much better I'm feeling from using this Colloidal Silver. I have more energy, and I just feel good. I only know that Dr. S is doing everything he can to help me, and I'm grateful! I'm not to sure about Dr. W. I haven't heard from him as of yet.

I slept good again. I can't wait to see Dr. S so we can see what's next to try.

He asked me to document how I feel and any changes I experience while on these natural treatments. I started using Calcium Lactate Powder (half a scoop in the morning and half a scoop in the evening). You mix it with water and drink it down.

Dr. W called and faxed me an instruction sheet for a colonoscopy.

I sure will be glad when this day is over. Carrie and Monet drove me up to the clinic and dropped me off. I signed the necessary forms and went back to get prepped. They wheeled me into the procedure room, where they placed a BP monitor and the IV into my arm. Dr. Y came in and discussed the procedure; we talked about Celiac disease, then the discussion started to heat up. I asked him about this colonoscopy for determining if I had Celiac's disease, and he told me, "Dr. L ordered this test because of all the cancer that runs in your family; this colonoscopy won't detect Celiac disease."

I said, "Why didn't you tell me this before when I was here in your office? Otherwise, I would have never had this colonoscopy test run!"

If I could have managed to get off the table, I would have dressed and called my daughter to come and get me. But by the time we were having this discussion, I was in an unconscious state. Before I knew it, Carrie and Monet were standing by my bedside. The nurse helped me get up and dressed, where we met in Dr. Y's office; he was beaming. No cancer or polyps. I'm upset and confused. Dave was really mad and said, "These doctors are doing it to you again. They have put you through the mill again and still no answers!" I know he's right, and he has every right to be angry over this. I fasted again this morning and went in for labs at Lab Corp. and not at the hospital. Lab Corp. was proud of me for standing up to Dr. Y about where I should go for my blood work. "You should have results by Friday," they told me. I'm still recovering from the colonoscopy and from being off my natural medicines and then going back on them. I went to Dr. S for a back treatment and to discuss these lesions. Dr. S told me to use chlorophyll on spots concentrating on my eating plan and detoxing. I rubbed the chlorophyll on my spots. The smell wasn't bad, but being the salve was green, I looked like Kermit the frog.

I'm feeling so much better, it's unbelievable! I am so thankful for Dr. S, I went to my therapy and just breezed through my exercise routines. Everyone was so happy to see me again at therapy; the other patients were all laughing and having a great time. I was walking on the treadmill, and my wrist was wrapped in a paraffin glove. I was laughing and probably walking too fast. I stepped a little off center and fell off the treadmill. There were four other patients in the vicinity of where I was who grabbed a hold of me before I passed out. They managed to get me on a chair, put an ice pack around my neck, and gave me a glass of juice while I sat and rested. This reminded me again of the "herxheimer reaction" that I have experienced a number of times in the past with the Lyme disease. I was a bit embarrassed, but they all made me feel good and were all concerned over what had taken place. I came home to rest; I was achy all over.

I called my friend who also has Lyme disease, trying to encourage her to come to Dr. S, but she's just not willing to give it a try. I suppose after all she's been through and how rudely she's been treated by the mainstream medical community she has a huge distrust of doctors.

I started coughing again. Cold? Allergy? I went to Dr. S for a treatment; I'm using mega doses of Calcium Lactate Powder and my silver hydrosol. I'm also sitting on my ice pack for the spinal stenosis; when I get my back treatments, sometimes it's a little aggressive so I just use ice to help with the inflammation. Dr. L ordered up blood work

Dr. S is concerned about my adrenal system. He put me on Ashawaganda, a tonic from the nightshade family and is particularly useful for a stressed patient. The next one is Rheumania; it detoxifies blood, liver, and kidneys. The third one is Licorice to treat skin, coughs, bronchitis, inflammation, arthritis, and it can also rid the lungs of mucus plus it's great for sore throats.[20]

I can't begin to tell you how wonderful these combinations of liquids are.

Dr. S commented on the Lyme disease and stated, "This disease is so deeply rooted in your cellular structure." He told me, "You need to stop stressing over everything!"

I had the kids over for dinner; then Monet and I played hide-and-seek. I was chasing her around the house when I felt a spell come over me, and I inadvertently knew I was going to fall down, so when I hit the floor I just lay there laughing.

I ended up with a knee brace. I haven't been to therapy for a while since I had taken a spell on the treadmill. The doctors weren't giving me a script to return; they are concerned about whether I'd pass out again.

My leg brace is on; my left foot where I had the fractures is hurting again. I don't understand why my body is in such turmoil. Then to top it off, Dr. L didn't do squat with my blood tests—no calcium or silver readings. I'm wondering if IDSA (Infectious Disease Society of America) isn't behind all of this. Because Lyme disease tests aren't all that definitive, I know I have the Lyme antibody in me, and I needed to know how active the Lyme disease is. I'm beginning to lose faith in my medical doctor. My knee is paining me badly; my left leg is just as painful, and I'm concerned about this lump in my neck. I wonder if I have an underactive thyroid or if my adrenal system is the problem.

I went to see Dr. L, and he scheduled me for an ultrasound for the lump in the base of my neck. He wanted to get to the bottom of my symptoms, due to the passing out, LBP/HBP, weight gain, and diarrhea. He then prescribed Ambien CR to help with my sleeplessness.

The neck lump was a swollen lymph node under my skin in my throat at the base of my neck. Dr. L felt it wasn't a cause for concern.

I'm having a tough time getting through the days and nights. The weather is snowy, and more snow is expected. I sat looking out the window over the fields that lay silent, covered with snow that glistened like a thousand diamonds spilt all across the field. Why do bad things happen to good people? I didn't allow my illness too happen; God has been right here beside me.

I'm praying that my immune system will withstand the flu or a cold. I'm not focusing on this lump in my neck either. I have been placed on many prayer chains, and I'm trusting that God will watch over me!

I sit here and worry about money, paying the bills on time, husband's working way too much and too hard, trying to meet the demands of his customers! I feel like such a burden for him, with all the medical bills, medical appointments,—never-ending confusion of having Lyme disease.

Both of my doctors gave me a lecture for worrying all the time. They said, "Your body is trying to tell you to slow down and regroup your thought processes. Listen to it!"

I told the ultrasound technician about the lump in my neck, so she placed this cold jelly on my throat and neck and placed a microphone over it, going from side to side and up and down.

After she did the test, I told her my prayer chains were praying for me. "Maybe all those prayers took it away," I said. She just looked at me and grinned and said, "Yes, wouldn't that be something?"

I had been researching Lyme disease for any new tests that were available. I received an e-mail from a Lyme disease patient in Connecticut; they went into the Plum Island Conspiracy Theory, an island in New York, about the lab and a huge article. I sometimes wonder if there's more truth to this than we realize and if this is why Lyme disease is so "hushed over" by so many of our mainstream medical community.

Then I discussed Plum Island with another sister of mine, and she didn't think I should be researching this topic.

The pain seems better, but I'm still given to tears! The pain just pounds at me; sometimes it's amazing how the weather can affect me, and the impact it has on my body is unbelievable. I am like my own weather station I can tell when a cold front or rain is approaching, I can feel it start in my muscles and my bones ache profusely. Then once it passes, I go back to my normal pain. I'm in so much pain I'm tempted to use a pain pill that my husband had from his eye surgery. I was afraid to use them because my BP is already low, and then it has a tendency to spike. I just used some Aleve, and throughout the day it slowly subsided.

While I was on the bike at therapy, the therapist couldn't locate my pulse. I sat down on a chair, and there was a student who was studying to be a physical therapist who assisted me trying to locate my pulse. She was pushing on my neck, sides of my neck, chest, and wrist when she finally found a very faint pulse. So I rested for a while, and then my hand was dipped into that warming hot paraffin, wrapped in saran wrap and nice warm towel so they could perform an ultrasound test on my wrist.

I went to Dr. S, and he performed an allergy treatment on me for virus and bacteria. He suggested that I put a drop or two of silver in my hands and snort the silver up into my nostrils. I know that sounds chaotic and even a bit strange, but it worked! When I called him about my earache, he said, "Take three or four drops put in the ear; tilt your head, place a cotton ball in, and do as needed."

I had my dream again of the bench. I have lost three brothers and an older sister and my parents. When I saw this bright light appear, it's beautiful and so peaceful, two of my brothers and my sister were smiling at me. Sometimes I think that my own departure from all of this will be coming sooner than I think. But I'm not ready, Lord! I have too much to do yet. I ask God to give me comfort and heal me of this devastating nightmare of Lyme disease and keep me safe so I can finish my work here on earth.

I am trying to stay focused, so I pray the Lord's prayer when I feel overwhelmed.

My earache is better; my throat isn't as sore and my cough seems to be much better as well. I can barely stand up without feeling as though I'm in a funhouse at the fair, everything is upside down and lopsided.

I had to call Dr. L so he could figure out why my ears are so plugged and what he could do to help me. I'm using natural alternatives with Dr. S to help me along with the Lyme disease because my body cannot take the conventional methods of treatment. But I also realize that there are times when I have to use conventional methods because nothing else seems to work for me. Yes, I'm ticked off!

I believe I have an ear infection in both ears. Both ears are totally plugged, and I can't hear a thing but the sound of my heart beating. I feel totally cut off from the world, but my husband has been very patient with me. He has to speak louder than usual; he puts the surround sound on in the living room so I can hear the TV.

My ears are starting to open up. Thank the good Lord for that! I went to see Dr. L for a follow-up on the lump in the base of my neck; thankfully again it was only soft tissue. So we are not going to worry over this situation anymore. He also placed me on a cancellation list for Dr. DR, the endocrinologist. I've been having a great deal of difficulty with weight gain, adrenal glands not functioning, dizziness, cold body temperatures, low blood pressure, and fainting.

I explained to him that I wasn't too thrilled with what he was wanting to give me to get the infection released from both of my ears. You see, the decadron injection is a steroid, and steroids in any form are a bad omen for chronic Lyme disease. It causes the Lyme disease to grow, but in my case when you get desperate for relief, you take routes you never dreamed of just to feel better.

As of right now, my right foot on the side where I had a wart removed is killing me. I can barely stand to put pressure on it when I walk. My left knee feels like it's out of out of joint once again. All this is of a great concern to me because I have been down this rocky road several times in the past twelve years. When I have developed all these symptoms and have so many tests involved, then to have all the tests return negative, it tells me one thing—that the Lyme disease is back in full swing, and even though I don't want to admit it to myself, I know what I'm going to have to do. I will need to return to Dr. J, my Lyme disease doctor, and schedule an appointment with him. This means that I will be back on an antibiotic again since we chronic Lyme disease patients have nothing else available on the market to use.

I've tried doing this naturally in an alternative state by using natural medications, vitamins, and supplements, but I know that Dr. S is going to be deeply hurt when I tell him his program is not working. I mean, let's face it, everything that I've taken with him, especially the new formulas, have worked; but chronic Lyme disease seems to be only controlled with aggressive rounds of antibiotics. The natural approach has helped my immune system beautifully, and I will probably still continue to use them to a point. I've been able to stay well so far by doing this.

Sometimes our bodies just build up immunity to natural supplements as well as conventional therapies. This is how it works with me. I have to take breaks in between and then start again and see what happens.

I have been using several vitamins and supplements for five years since I went to Dr. S. He has never steered me off course, although many skeptics think it's a little overboard. It's amazing when I stop to think about how much or how many vitamins I consume everyday, all day.

If symptoms persist despite antibiotic use, there may be an on-going infection requiring further treatment. This can include months and even years of oral or intravenous antibiotics or a combination of antibiotics. Long term antibiotic therapy is needed because B.Burgdorferi becomes dormant and hides within the cells. Our immune systems are terribly affected by all of this and thus it creates a long time to clear toxins from our bodies. Natural alternative medicine approaches it differently natural therapy wants to enhance the immune system. I feel personally that using antibiotic therapy along with natural alternative supplements has made a huge difference in my slow recovery. It amazes me how backward we are in the United States when it comes to healthcare and how surrounding countries are so much more advanced and further ahead on treating diseases. Lyme is a tremendously debilitating disease. I know for a fact that using the normal approach of antibiotics and the alternative natural way has worked well for me. If anything at all, it has given me an empowerment of self-awareness to take my healthcare into my own hands.Most chronic Lyme disease patients will try just about anything to feel better and to somehow function. Not all chronic Lyme disease patients are willing to resolve to these drastic measures; it's not an insurable coverage from the insurance companies, it's all out of pocket expenses.

I have spent thousands of dollars in the past five years; fortunately with my husband's help and my disability I have been able to afford to do this. But this was my choice, and no matter by what means, I will continue to do so. Because it has given me more time to enjoy life a little more, to have energy to be a part of my husband's life, my children's lives, and my granddaughter's childhood. And to me if this buys me more time for them, then it has been worth it all!

But it also scares me to death that if I stop using the natural medications and go back to the conventional method of treating chronic Lyme disease, how long will I hold up? I feel like a time bomb just waiting for someone to pull the detonator! I do believe my immune system has gained some momentum, and so maybe I can continue with Dr. S's protocol while I'm on the antibiotic for the chronic Lyme disease.

My mother-in-law is seventy-six. God love her, I've had to depend on her many a day to take me to the doctor as well. I can't drive right now because I can't hear! It's not easy being dependent on others, but as I've said before, thank God we have loved ones or someone to help with our burdens along the way. It also goes back to letting others help you; there's no shame in asking for help.

For many years while I was dealing with chronic Lyme disease when I was unable to do for myself, I believe it was more difficult for me to ask for help. Even my friends and some family members made me feel embarrassed about asking or needing help with everyday activities or household duties. When I was unable to hold a job down, that realization hit me like a rock; and not only that, all the money that was scattered into the wind through the incompetent mainstream medical community that my husband and I spent on, for what? Such a wasteful amount of lost time and heartache that they caused me, lost hours, days, weeks, months and even years I'll never get back!

I was approached many times on getting assistance through a lawyer who represented Lyme disease patients in the area. I was shocked that anyone would suggest that to me, and I felt defeated and degraded because of it. How can I face my friends and family knowing that I, at forty-eight years old, should need disability, and little did I know what and how long it would take for my lawyer to fight for me to receive SSD.

My ears are slowly opening up, I can't imagine what silence would be like forever.

I went to Dr. S, and he checked my ears; the right ear is much worse than the left ear. He is very disappointed with the natural treatment; he felt sure that the silver and the calcium would knock these infections on its heels. He adjusted my back and my knee. He worked on my ears. He grabbed both of my earlobes—first the left and the right lobe twisted and pulled down on them; then he rubbed with two fingers on each side of my neck below my ears to open the airways. He instructed me to rub them every hour for the rest of the day and the night. I thought this to be weird, but the results were amazing.

Dr. S did acupressure on my earlobes again; he jerked them, and I couldn't believe how they cracked. I never knew your earlobes would crack. I discussed the adrenogen I'd been using for my adrenal system and how it gave me heartburn, so Dr. S did an allergy treatment against the adrenogen.

If you didn't know any better, you might think Dr. S was a witch doctor. He does some pretty amazing treatments, and he knows so many things to make you feel better; surprisingly, they all work! I am so blessed, I wish my brother Tommy was here so I could personally thank him for steering me to Dr. S, what a God-send this doctor is and will continue to be. I slept really great last night.

Dr. S ran an allergy treatment for the Iso D-3, which is Vitamin D, and this also cleared. As I said before, some of us Lyme disease patients will try just about anything to alleviate pain. I was researching a site about detoxing foot patches. Detoxion foot patches are the rage of Asia; detoxion is an all-natural patch that amazingly extracts heavy metals and other forms of toxins from your system while you sleep. First it contains tourmaline, which is a mineral found in Brazil. It passes a unique property of emitting infrared rays FIR, which generates negative ions.

When worn on your foot (bottom of your foot), the negative ions stimulate acupressure meridian points for various vital organs, which promote improved circulation and detoxification. Secondly, detoxion contains a wood vinegar essence from bamboo that has an amazing ability to absorb toxins through your skin.[21]

I was so excited to go to bed. I couldn't wait to sleep just so morning would come, and I could see the results. I slept good all night. When I woke up the following morning, I couldn't believe what I saw on those foot pads. They were black and green, moist, and it was gross, but I figured they must be working.

I went to Dr. S and gave him a copy of Detoxion, and he was very anxious for me as to what the results may show. He manipulated my lower back and neck, and then he was looking at the lesions on my arm. I told him they were improving.

I wore my foot patches again, and they were black and green, yuck! Then I realized I had put my detox foot pads on wrong; they were upside down, and when I woke up the next morning they were still white.

I went to see Dr. S, and he was amused by all of this. He said, "The pain you are having is not from detoxing. Detoxing doesn't cause pain; it helps to rid your body of toxins. You have to remember, Janet, it's not just the Lyme disease you are dealing with." Again, Dr. S is correct!

I placed my foot detox pads on my feet again (correctly); when I woke up and took them off they were black and grey. The detox foot pads made me feel warm and tingly all over; I had some energy, and I was a little calmer.I decided to take the foot pads and place them on my ankles. It helped some, but I'd better just use them for the soles of my feet.

I'm trying to stay focused. I was reading my Daily Bread about cheering each other on. If you have nothing else to give, you can give encouragement. I must keep my eyes to the Lord for his strength and help. I can't depend on anyone but Him!

One evening we were watching TV, and they had a piece on these foot detox pads, telling people that they aren't any good. Of course, I knew that when something works, there's always someone putting it down. The news media and the pharmaceutical companies do not want the public to use these items for fear of hurting their pocketbooks. It's all about the money!

I am noticing improvements by using these foot detox pads, and I differ with the news media. I have had several comments from skeptics, but I also have had many compliments on how much better I was looking.

I become very emotional over Lyme disease when I feel that I need to defend the disease in skeptical eyes who do not know the recourse of what I've had to deal with in twelve years. I have a right to stand my ground and speak up for myself and for other Lyme disease victims who can't or who are afraid to speak up. I'm not, and I will do everything in my power to take a necessary stand for Lyme disease.

Campaigning:

TAKING ON WASHINGTON, DC

I have been campaigning for Lyme disease, writing letters to Congress, sending emails to Lyme disease patients; it's time consuming and wears on my mind and makes me physically exhausted and mentally drained.

AUG. 17, 2007

We still haven't determined why I have been passing out. The doctor's seem to have shoved me under the rug, go figure! I wonder if it's due to the controversy of the Lyme disease with the infectious disease society and all their ridiculous protocols.

Daryl Hall of Hall & Oates, a music group, has Lyme disease. In July of 2005 he woke up feeling like he had a bad case of the flu. He was right in the middle of a show when his body gave out. He ended up cancelling his tour to recover from what he thought was the flu. His ex-girlfriend advised him to get diagnosed for

Lyme disease because she has it also. He then found Dr. B, a well-known controversial and literate Lyme disease doctor. In 2001, NY States Administration Review Board for Professional Conduct brought a case against this medical doctor for medical negligence. The charges were for prescribing long-term antibiotic therapy for Lyme disease, unfortunately this doctor is now retired!

This is such a disgrace and discriminating abscess that so many Lyme disease literate physicians are subjected to.

It's assumed that President George W. Bush caught Lyme disease while vacationing in Kennebunkport, Maine. It was announced that he'd been treated for Lyme disease the previous year. August 13, 2007 at 4:10pm from The Guardian in the United Kingdom, this is public knowledge, it was on the news. The White House reported last week that President Bush was treated for Lyme disease last summer after he discovered the bulls eye rash associated with the disease on his leg. Given the controversy that surrounds the disease it is difficult to see why Bush would not disclose his treatment. If our suspicions are true, this is yet another disgusting episode of this administration's hypocrisy. He personally has benefitted from a course of treatment that through his silence he would deny to tens of thousands of others.

My attitude, determination, optimism, constant prayers to God for strength, and the love and support of my husband and my family has helped me come full circle with living with Lyme disease. I have learned to accept what I have; I have learned to live with Lyme disease, I found doctors that have helped me whether conventional or naturally. I am getting on with living, trying to go out and be a blessing for others who are suffering and to make a difference!

The vigilance and determination to find doctors out there who have and are continuing to serve me in every way possible has given me hope. This is such a huge impact on my fight for survival—to keep going no matter what!

I wrote a letter to one of the medical doctors on the Infectious Disease Society Board and asked him why we can't get Lyme disease recognized. Why is it that when Lyme disease is mentioned to a physician or anyone in the medical field, they look at us like we have leprosy?

This disease has cost me dearly. My husband could live life a bit easier now if a Lyme literate doctor could have helped me twelve years ago. I've lost friendships and some of my family members who do not fully understand how this disease affects me. Thankfully, my husband has stood by my side and supported me to keep fighting. I feel very blessed because I know of many marriages that have been broken from having a spouse with Lyme disease.

No one wants to listen to me and to millions of us who have suffered needlessly at the hands of the mainstream medical community. The Infectious Disease Society is taking away our voices, our rights, and our freedoms. Many chronic Lyme disease patients are losing their doctors; they can't get insurance coverage or are being denied with their insurance they already have.

The IDSA, insurance carriers, and the medical community want to point fingers at those who suffer daily with chronic Lyme disease and then deny us from getting medical attention.

I wrote a letter in May of 2008 to our local congressman. Part of my letter is below:

I'm sure you are aware of the controversy surrounding Lyme disease and the House Bill HR741 on the House Health Subcommittee Agenda.

The IDSA and their ridiculous guidelines for diagnosis and treatment protocols is in the process of denying Lyme disease patients of a chance for a bill to be passed in IDSA's favor and not ours (Lyme disease).

Lyme disease is a serious bacterial infection that develops from an infected tick. The disease is often misdiagnosed and goes untreated for years in many victims. In my case, has proven to be a devastating, expensive, chronic health condition. I feel it is irresponsible for doctors too simply ignore Lyme disease. I have suffered as millions of Lyme disease patients have and still are with persistent health problems, neurological disorders, crippling muscle and joint pain, disabling fatigue, psychological disorders, and even death in some cases.

Lyme disease has cost me thousands of dollars wasted, lost time with my family and friends, lost time that I will never get back.

No one wants to listen to our pleas for help.

Lyme disease needs to be recognized. We need more reliable testing procedures and the public and the news media need to be educated and our doctors here in Ohio and other states need to be educated and given the opportunity to treat Lyme disease patients without fear that IDSA or Medical Conduct Boards may shut them down.

Lyme disease it is a real disease just like any other. It makes me sick that Lyme disease victims cannot get this disease recognized for what it truly is.

We need this HR741 on the House Health Subcommittee Agenda today. Congressman, I am asking for your help and understanding.

I did receive a very nice letter from the congressman.

> Thank you very much for writing me with your concerns. I appreciate your taking the time to share your views with me. Hearing from you is both important and helpful because it provides me with insight into your thoughts and concerns on the major issues we face today as a nation and especially as Ohioans. You can be certain that I will give your concerns my full consideration as the legislative process continues.

I received an e-mail from the Portland Independent Media Center that the United States government admits that Lyme disease is a bio weapon. The existence of the Lyme disease epidemic is officially covered up; its myriads of misdiagnoses from Lupus to MS to hypochondria is astounding, to say the least.

Plum Island in *Poison Plum* is a virtual hotbed to some of the deadliest germs that's ever roamed the earth. Plum Island is marked red or yellow, and it's a highly restricted location for dangerous animal diseases. It is a biological time bomb!

The thought of this makes me sick and somewhat scared have to death to think that our government would create this to incapacitate citizens or to even destroy our nation. What has happened to the United States of America?

Is this why, when Lyme disease is mentioned, the mainstream medical community shove it under the carpet or dispute it? Why is it so controversial? Is Lyme disease a genetically engineered disease that either leaked out, or was it a deliberate stance for population control? I feel, as do many others, that Lyme is very political!

The morals are falling by the wayside, and I don't just mean the morals of our citizens. I'm talking about the morals of our government and how can these congressman and congresswomen sleep at night knowing all this.

All I can say for now is the battle for me with chronic Lyme disease isn't over yet! It is a continual battle. I have come a long way in twelve years, but I know I have a long way's to go to recover. I will continue to be vigilant, researching, studying and praying to God for continued strength and devotion. I will continue on with Dr. S and my other wonderful medical doctors and Lyme disease doctor if necessary. I will keep a sense of humor, sense of balance in my life the music will continue to flow from my heart. I will continue to keep using the natural alternatives for my healthcare or until the Lyme disease decides to end my life.

Writing this book was extremely difficult, mind boggling, and exhausting. Not in a million years would I have ever thought of writing a book. It was a difficult journey for me, but I am so grateful to have had the opportunity to accomplish such a task. So no matter what your circumstances are or whatever fate has dealt you, you can do it! Look at me, I did!

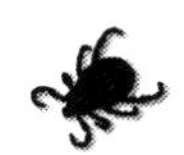

Bibliography

www.ICHTherapy.com

www. Deepforest208485@aol.com

www.aldf.com/deertickecology

www.sciencedaily.com

www.turnthecorner.org/tick-borne diseases, Oct. 26, 2006

www.doctorofhomeopathy.com

www.cyberbohemia.com/Pages/history sweat lodge

www.ohionaturopathic.com

www.webmd.com

www.spring4health.com

Traficant, HR2790, The Lyme disease Initiative 2000, 6–5

Assoc.content/health&wellness/Lyme disease

Bull's-eye Vol. 9.5 Sept. 1999

Auto Immunity, *The Common Thread* by Noel Rose, MD & PHD

A travel guide to heaven by Anthony DeStefano

Ruth Graham, A legacy of love

Energy Times July/August 2008

The tapestry of healing

Power of Prayerful Living by Doug Hill-God take this pain by Marianne Williamson

Joyce Meyer's

Detoxion Ionic foot patch by Holistec

www.birdssuite101.com/article

www.checkmd.com

www.picclinenursing.com

www.en.wikipedia.org/Lymedisease

www.allhealth.com

www.familydoctor.org

www.esciencenews.com

www.merck.com

www.canlyme.org

www.Lymediseaseresearchdatabase.com

www.clinicaltrials.gov

www.lymebook.com/Africa.europe-canada-sweden-england-unitedkingdom

www.peteducation.com

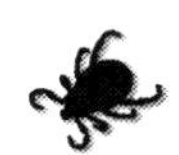

Endnotes

1 (Bull's-eye Vol. 9.5 Sept. 1999)

2 (Animal Health from Fort Dodge, Iowa)

3 (www.doublecheckmd.com).

4 (www.picclinenursing.com).

5 Jerry Baker, Great Green Book of Garden Secrets, 2000

6 (www.allhealth.com)

7 Robynns_Lyme_List@YahooGroups.com6 Westbank, BC Canada)

8 www.Lymediseaseresearchdatabase.com.

9 Clinicaltrials.gov is a site you can go to for evaluation, treatment, and follow-up for patients with Lyme disease. This is verified by the National Institutes of Health Clinical Center (CC) August 2009.

10 (www.ICHTherapy.com)

11 (Newsweek Article Sept. 17, 2000 from deepforest208485@aol.com)

12 (Traficant, HR2790, The Lyme disease Initiative 2000, June 5)

13 (Energy Times July/August 2008)

14 www.Allnurses.com

15 (www.ohionaturopathic.com)

16 The Power of Prayerful Living Pg.435 on Battling Depression in Rodale Press 2001

17 (Natural-Immunogenics. Corp.) www.sovereignsilver.info

18 (www.spring4health.com)

19 Susan Umphress and Marilyn Nelson, Twice An Angel: Living and Dying with Lyme Disease

20 (www.naturalherbsguide.com 2/19/09)

21 (Detoxion Ionic Foot Patch Distributed by Holistec)